Peter Mark Adams

THE HEALING FIELD

Energy, Consciousness and Transformation

BALBOA.
PRESS

A DIVISION OF HAY HOUSE

Balboa Press books may be ordered through booksellers or by contacting:

Balboa Press
A Division of Hay House
1663 Liberty Drive
Bloomington, IN 47403
www.balboapress.com
1 (877) 407-4847

Printed in the United States of America.

ISBN: 978-1-4525-8356-3 (sc)
ISBN: 978-1-4525-8358-7 (hc)
ISBN: 978-1-4525-8357-0 (e)

Library of Congress Control Number: 2013918164

Balboa Press rev. date: 1/14/2014

Acknowledgements

A very special thanks to Yesim Cimcoz for being a supportive friend and a great writing coach during the long process of researching, writing and reworking this text. Thanks are also due to all those healers who freely shared their knowledge and experiences with me and to all the people who offered accounts of their private experiences. Many thanks to Michael & Richard Greenwood for allowing me to use one of their illustrations. Last, but not least, a very special thanks to my wife, life partner and a great healer, Gülcan Arpacıoğlu-Adams, for providing many of the healing cases that I have used in this book. Thanks also for all of her patience and support during the long process of researching and writing this book.

For Gülcan

Contents

Illustrations

Introduction

The Healing Field arose from a prolonged meditation on the diverse ways in which we experience healing and personal transformation. I have been lucky enough to undertake this journey in the company of my wife, Gulcan, and many other gifted healers and psychics who provided unstinting help and guidance. In the process I witnessed wonders that revealed a greatly expanded conception of self, reality and our place within it. I found myself asking why it is that these things are so little known, so rarely experienced and so obscured from view. Because many of these experiences possessed such rare and unusual qualities I wanted to share them since they suggest a far more expansive and uplifting view of whom and what we are than mainstream thinking allows for.

This book will help to illuminate these issues by dwelling upon those aspects of reality that are most controversial, most challenging and difficult to find. Although this work is anchored in science, its subject matter occupies that twilight zone between objective science and subjective experience, between reason and intuition. All of the anomalous phenomena dealt with here are backed up by the records of our own case files and, as far as possible, by the available scientific research. Above all I wanted to facilitate an understanding of the larger web of life and of our place within it. For when we grasp this, we begin to move towards a quality of understanding that relieves much of the fear, doubt and uncertainty that overshadows the vast majority of people.

The Healing Field has been structured to progress from the day to day anomalies that most of us have experience of towards the more unusual and, in some cases, disturbing phenomena that occur on the outermost edges of human experience. For it is only by examining the full range of such experiences that we can grasp the hidden depths of reality and the true expanse of the human spirit. In Chapter 1, 'Healing, energy and consciousness', we set the scene by introducing the main categories and issues that we are going to deal with. In Chapter 2, 'Psi and intuitive perception', we look at how each and every one of us has the dynamic potential to access information with which we have no connection. In Chapter 3, 'Healing issues within our time-line', we examine experiences from the extremities of our normal lifecycle: those arising in the womb, during the birth process and on the very brink of death. These experiences challenge the conventional understanding of consciousness and the boundaries of selfhood, of when 'we' can be said to exist. In Chapter 4, 'Healing issues beyond our time-line', we extend our inquiry into the continuity of the self and the limits of consciousness by examining examples of healing involving past lives as well as inherited family and ancestral trauma. Chapter 5, 'The healing field', summarizes the implications of what we have learned up to now and proposes a model of consciousness and reality that allows us to make sense of these otherwise anomalous experiences. In Chapter 6, 'Healing on extended planes', we expand our horizon once more to examine healing on levels of reality beyond the range of our immediate perceptual awareness. We consider the role of entity attachments of varying degrees of sentience that act to affect our health and mental balance. Chapter 7, 'Healing through spirit', considers mystical or 'peak experiences', the variety of ways in which these are accessed and how they contribute to healing and the ethical and spiritual development of humanity. Finally, in

Chapter 8, 'Conclusions', we pull all of this material together to develop an understanding of consciousness, reality and identity that incorporates these phenomena. We use this model to suggest strategies that will lead to profound levels of healing, increased happiness and a greater contribution to spiritual coevolution.

Chapter 1

Healing, energy & consciousness

Introducing Healing, Energy and Consciousness

Ten years ago I was diagnosed by a medical doctor and acupuncturist with an enlarged liver. His diagnosis involved using a micro ohm-meter to monitor variations in the skin's electrical resistance on the main acupuncture meridian points. He told me that my condition could be healed but this would require weekly treatments for the next 8 months. A day or so later my wife, Gulcan, and I met a Russian bioenergist who offered to demonstrate her healing skills. Since neither of us shared a common language we couldn't discuss my health issues, or anything else for that matter. Instead she passed her hands around me at a short distance from my body and quickly diagnosed the same liver condition as the acupuncturist. This impressed me, and I decided to undertake a healing session with her the following week. The session started with her bringing her own energy into 'focus'. She asked me to breathe deeply and rapidly a few times. I am familiar with various sorts of breathwork so I recognized that this would quickly increase the level of my inner energy. She then massaged my liver, and this marked the last second at which my awareness could be said to be operating within normal bounds. She inhaled sharply. As she did so her hands pulled some manner of 'blockage' from my liver as though she was ripping a plant, roots and all, out of the soil. I distinctly felt 'it' move from me to her. She then exhaled powerfully over my head. Right then my whole mood and energy shifted. I felt weak and light at the same time. Although these actions describe what happened, they completely fail to do justice to the intensity of the process that I experienced.

When she 'pulled' the problem out and into herself it showed quite clearly in the pain and sadness that were etched into her face. A moment later she lifted her face upwards and powerfully blew out, permanently and completely releasing the problem. I felt weak. I lay down. All of a sudden I was completely overcome by what I can only describe as ecstatic bliss, pure and endless joy, a sense of the unutterable, perfection and humor of existence itself. I dissolved in joyful laughter – a level and depth of laughter that I have never experienced before. I laughed uncontrollably for half an hour. About a week later, I visited the acupuncturist who checked my liver once more only to find, much to his amazement, that he could no longer find any trace of the liver problem. When we told him about my session with the bioenergist he said, "I must meet this woman!" Ten years later I am still completely free of the liver problem.

This account touches on many of the themes that we will be exploring through the first-hand accounts of gifted energy healers. In particular it illustrates the intimate connection that exists between our natural energy fields, our health and the quality of our awareness. It demonstrates our innate ability to intuitively understand the deep, emotional roots of ill health. And it shows how natural processes can affect fast and effective healing by changing the dynamics of our energy field.

The reality revealed through energy based healing is quite different from the world of most people's day to day experience. Like most of us, I have been raised to believe that what you see is all there is and everything in the universe can be reduced to and explained by particles of matter bumping into one another. But the accounts of healing gathered here, drawn for the most part from our own case files, reveal that this picture is grossly inadequate. Reality is far more complex, multidimensional and connected than we imagine. Each and every one of us, using only natural methods, can realize a level of healing and positive personal transformation far beyond conventional expectations.

Like everyone else I possess an in-built skepticism to any suggestion that reality is fundamentally different from what my day to day experience, or mainstream science, tells me. When challenged by anomalies that exceed this one-size-fits-all worldview, the response is usually one of ridicule, outright dismissal or rationalization.

There are very good reasons why a change in our worldview is long overdue. People are increasingly aware, and accepting the fact, that their experience does not accord with mainstream science. Recently, one of the world's leading philosophers, Thomas

Nagel, triggered a storm of criticism by stating the obvious fact that the 500 year old scientific project of attempting to explain everything in terms of interactions amongst the smallest particles, called reductive materialism, has failed[1]. A similar point had been made by the biologist and complexity theorist Stuart Kauffman[2]. It has failed because it cannot account for the most defining and essential features of life: consciousness, agency, meaning and values. By 'consciousness' we mean the irreducible, luminous awareness of the present moment shared by all sentient beings. It is sometimes hard to grasp, but this dynamic quality that so essentially defines us, escapes all explanation, whether on the part of philosophy, neuroscience, psychology or evolutionary theory. By 'agency' we refer to the fundamental quality of intentionality that all sentient beings possess: our desiring, willing, planning and executing. Purposeful action gives rise to meaning, another fundamental quality of being. And with meaningful action come values. Values capture our inherent sensitivity towards such fundamental issues as right and wrong and justice and injustice. We all know that these essential elements are characteristic of all sentient life and form an intrinsic part of reality. And yet, modern science can find no place for them. Where we find these qualities at their most pronounced is in the arena of healing, personal and spiritual transformation. For this reason we need to remain open to the possibility that anomalous experiences in these contexts, such as those that accompanied my own healing, may well be pointing us towards a broader conception of reality and consciousness than has been accepted up to now.

The process by which we come to hold our beliefs about the nature of reality, consciousness and personal identity, our enculturation or 'programming', prepares us to 'fit in' with a certain society and culture. But just because it enables us to interact with the portion of reality relevant to our society doesn't mean that it also prepares us for perceiving those aspects of reality beyond our society's sphere of interest. For this, we require a different point of view, new concepts, language and a fresh understanding and approach to the familiar world we inhabit. I liken this process to 'deprogramming'.

My own 'de-programming' has been a continuing process over many years. One event that helped me occurred when I was growing up in Africa in the early 1960s. We had driven from the Kenyan highlands down through the Rift Valley and then south east. All day we travelled on the rough red earth road that, in those years, ran all the way to the coast. We crossed dried-up riverbeds and vast tracks of featureless savannah, a great plume of red dust flowing out behind the car. Late that day we arrived on the edge of the city of Mombasa. We stopped at a small open market next to the road to pick up some fruit before going on to our final destination much further to the south. As we got out of the car a man stepped forward and warmly greeted Pedro, who was travelling with us. It was his brother. We asked Pedro how on earth his brother could possibly be waiting for him at such a remote place on that day and time. He shrugged, "Because I would be here" he said. In the early 1960s the internet and mobile phones were still 25 years or so in the future. And even supposing he had phoned sometime before we set off, it still doesn't explain his brother being at that particular roadside market at that time and our spontaneous decision to stop there. Is there more to reality than we can possibly imagine? As we explore the various cases presented here, we will see that the answer is a resounding 'yes'.

Another event that helped me to remain open to new possibilities occurred in my teens. I had joined a Karate club run by a highly respected Master, Ronnie Colwell. One night Ronnie demonstrated the controlled use of Chi energy. He had a few of the burlier club members hold three thick wooden boards – each around 12 inches (30 cm) square and around 2.5 inches (6.4 cm.) thick – tightly together. He then struck the first board – and nothing happened. But when we examined the boards we found that whilst the first and second boards showed no sign of damage the third board, the one furthest away from the strike, was neatly split down the middle. How he did this, how it was even possible, puzzled most of us at the time. It still does today, over 40 years later! The martial artist's explanation is that it is done by focusing their 'Chi' energy on a point beyond where they are going to strike. In this case Ronnie focused his energy on and split the third board, the one furthest away from the struck surface.

The reality of Chi energy and of our wider energy fields is apparent to those who practice the martial arts, the many forms of spiritual yoga or any of the energy based healing modalities. We will return to consider the nature of these energies and the evidence for them later. For now let's agree to call the energy surrounding all sentient beings 'biofield energy' to distinguish it from the conventional forms of electromagnetic energy produced by every organ and part of our bodies.

As we saw in my own case of healing, a gifted healer can intuitively access a deeper, more perceptive understanding of health problems than would be apparent to most of us. We describe the possession of such 'perceptual' skills as psychic ability. This is just one manifestation of a range of capabilities subsumed under the concept of 'Psi'. Because of the centrality of these abilities to many types of healing process we will examine them in greater detail in the next chapter. The insights that arise because of a healer's innate psychism, or Psi abilities, involve shifting awareness beyond the normal range of waking states. Such shifts are commonly called 'altered states of consciousness' (ASC).

Altered States of Consciousness

In every society and in every age, people have engaged in practices that shift their awareness to take in a much broader spectrum of reality. In the West we call these shifts 'altered states' and, until fairly recently, we have tended to dismiss them as psychological distortions or even as pathological. But in many societies, and amongst those dedicated to a broad range of healing and spiritual development practices, these shifts, and the realities they provide access to, form a vital part of everyday life. Our capacity to sense things hidden from normal perception is far more dynamic than many of us imagine.

The expression 'altered states of consciousness' was coined by psychologists and anthropologists in the 1960s to categorize the much broader range of experience reported by researchers, especially amongst nonWestern societies. Altered states were initially defined as any state that exhibited 'sufficient deviation'[3], a 'qualitative shift'[4] or 'difference'[5] from 'normal waking consciousness'. But definitions like this beg the question: what constitutes 'sufficient' and who is to judge what is 'normal'? Not only definitions like these, but the very need for such a category has been challenged by people from cultures who still utilize a much fuller spectrum of awareness. A Native American challenged the Transpersonal Psychologist on precisely this point,

> "I don't understand why you use the term 'non-ordinary states'. For my people, these experiences are part of the normal spectrum of human experience!"[6].

In some ways the idea of 'altered states' tells us more about the limitations our own culture than it does about the states themselves. States of consciousness, such as the various levels of wakefulness and sleep or certain meditative states, are relatively discrete. They can be identified by their 'signature' patterns of brain waves (Alpha, Beta etc.) and the activation of specific areas of the brain. But we cannot say the same for 'altered states'. The term does not identify any specific subjective experience or brain state. What, then, does it signify? It can, of course, cover anything from psychosis to drunkenness. But in general usage an 'altered state' designates an extension or expansion of awareness that fulfills some specific purpose. In other words, the significance of altered states lies not in the neuroscience, psychology or anthropology surrounding them, but in what they can do for us. Altered states provide alternative ways of engaging with reality. In all times and cultures altered states have been used to provide access to information and realities not accessible by other means, to facilitate healing and as an integral part of personal and spiritual transformation.

There are four basic contexts in which we see such shifts occurring: gaining access to remote information, healing, shamanism and mysticism. None of these areas excludes the others and they all exhibit a large degree of overlap. I have further characterized states of awareness that access remote information as transpersonal. This means that they are used to pick up information about distant, hidden or lost people and events. I have characterized most of the healing, shamanic and mystical states as transformational since they often accompany or even induce profound healing, personal and spiritual change.

As we noted, many skilled healers intuitively access unconscious, forgotten or hidden information that provides the key to their client's healing. These healers combine access to such information with other skills that facilitate the integration of emotional upsets and traumas. Some of the more exotic examples include fetal, birth related, ancestral and past life traumas. Practicing shaman combine Psi and healing skills with additional capabilities for working with a range of etheric, astral, non-human and other-dimensional 'entities'. Finally, mystics may combine all of these capabilities with a capacity for realizing and sustaining transcendent levels of awareness.

To provide context, we will use these categories to relate altered states to the more usual range of experiences, such as the various levels of wakefulness and sleep, and a few of the various classes of mental disorder. The idea is not to create an exhaustive classification of every possible state of consciousness, an impossible undertaking, but rather to provide a model that helps us to orientate ourselves to this complex material. Finally, we can add some of the experiences typically associated with each of these states as depicted in Diagram I (below).

Diagram I: The Spectrum of Consciousness

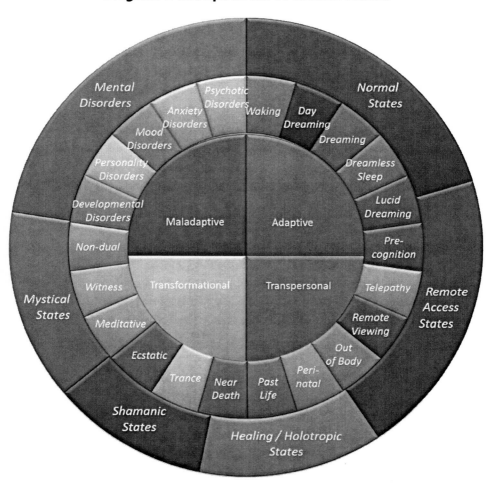

Notes

1. *Nagel, T. (2012) Mind and Cosmos: Why the Materialist Neo-Darwinian Conception of Nature is Almost Certainly False*

2. *Kauffman, S. (2008) Reinventing the Sacred: A New View of Science, Reason, and Religion*

3. *Ludwig, AM. 'Altered States of Consciousness' Journal of General Psychiatry (1966): 225*

4. *Tart, C. (editor) (1969) 'Altered States of Consciousness: A Book of Readings'*

5. *Krippner, S. 'Altered States of Consciousness' in J. White (Editor) (1972) The Highest State of Consciousness (p. 1-5).*

6. *Ehrmann, W. 'Some Critical Issues in Stan & Christina Grof's Holotropic Breathwork: A discussion between Wilfried Ehrmann, & Stan Grof M.D.' The Healing Breath, Vol. 3, No. 3, 2001*

Chapter 2

Psi & intuitive knowledge

Introducing Intuitive Knowledge

My wife, Gulcan, woke up one morning and said, "I can't stop thinking of Nursel. She's a friend of mine who moved to Canada. I haven't heard from her for nearly seven years. Her name is continuously on my mind. " At odd times throughout the day she repeated this and remarked that she was waiting for some development related to her. Sure enough, that afternoon she called Gulcan. She was in town and wished to meet up.

Although such experiences form a normal part of everyday life, especially in the context of close relationships, conventional thinking is unwilling to reflect upon their implications for our understanding of consciousness and reality. In fact, we are positively encouraged to dismiss them as mere 'coincidences'. But anything that regularly works to produce actionable knowledge cannot be dismissed so easily. Our thinking falls far short of many people's day to day experience.

We all possess an innate capability for Psi – the capacity to access information or influence events beyond the reach of our five senses. Such information may relate to the unknown past, lost or hidden objects and, though with many complications, the probability of certain future events. Most of us experience this capability as a sudden insight that breaks into the day to day flow of our thoughts. It often occurs when we least expect it, especially when we are in a relaxed de-focalized state of awareness. In such states we are far more open to registering emergent ideas and feelings. However, this kind of intuitive perception can also be deliberately induced. This is usually achieved through a combination of focusing on a specific piece of information and combining this with an otherwise relaxed and receptive state of mind.

The usual names for these various types of Psi are: premonition, precognition, retrocognition, clairvoyance and telepathy. Premonition is an emotional awareness of a 'future event'. Precognition is knowledge of such an event. Retrocognition is knowledge of an unknown past event. Clairvoyance is the perception of objects or events that are beyond the reach of our immediate senses. Telepathy is picking up information from another person, or sentient being, without sensory communication. Just how widespread are these phenomena?

Most people have experienced at least one of them at some time in their lives. Over half the US and European populations claim to have experienced telepathy, clairvoyance or contact with the dead. Though only a small percentage of people, around 10%, claim to have experienced all three. Overall more women than men report having these experiences but other factors, such as education, are irrelevant[1]. A further survey found that two thirds of the US population claim to have had a Psi or 'mystical' experience. Intriguingly, the incidence of these experiences is increasing with each successive generation[2].

The frequency with which people experience such events varies enormously. Some people make a living from their Psi related skills, others may have these experiences on almost a daily basis and still others hardly ever, if at all. There appear to be many different factors at work. As with most activities, innate talent is important but our openness to such possibilities and how we choose to develop our awareness are also crucial. If we are constantly absorbed in focused, and especially analytic, activity, we will tend to lack the receptivity for picking up more subtle indications.

Premonition & Precognition

One evening my wife and I had been eating out. After leaving the restaurant we crossed the road to do some window shopping shoes and bags as I recall! As I was waiting for her I was suddenly overcome by a sense of foreboding. I looked around the street and back across at the restaurant but nothing was happening. I felt puzzled. A minute later a figure slipped out of an alley next to the restaurant and threw a something onto its open terrace. There was a loud bang followed by the sound of breaking glass and people screaming. Luckily no one was hurt, though many people were in a state of shock. We went over and helped out. We then understood that it had only been a sound bomb and not something far worse.

Premonition is an emotional reaction to or awareness of a future event. Precognition is knowledge of such an event. Commonsense tells us that since future events do not exist yet, we cannot possibly be aware of them. Before we deal with this objection let's look at some of the available evidence and then return to consider the implications of it for our understanding of reality.

A standard experiment to test for premonition involves monitoring a subject's physiological responses to a series of randomly generated images. The images can be anything from soothing nature scenes to scenes of violence and death. In a statistically significant number of cases the physiological reactions appropriate to disturbing images are registered a few seconds before the image is actually shown. In fact, the physiological reaction to the disturbing image occurs a few seconds before the computer has even chosen which image to display. A recent review of nine experiments that tested for this effect concluded that all of the experiments except one confirmed our ability to be 'preaware' of something that may affect us negatively[3]. These results confirm those from a whole series of similar studies carried out over the last 15 years[4,5,6,7]. We, and presumably other animals, can be emotionally 'pre-aware' of lurking dangers if we are receptive to subtle nuances in our own feelings and physiology.

A range of experiments relating to premonition have been undertaken by the biologist Rupert Sheldrake. One famous experiment involved pets who seem to know when their owners are returning home. Even with trips of up to 15 kilometers from home and with a randomly selected return time, pets seem to know both when the owner decides to go back home and when their return journey actually starts. The percentage of their time waiting at a window in anticipation of their owner's return increases proportionately. It jumps from around 15% of their time normally to 25% during the 10 minutes or so when the decision to return is being made and up to 55% of their time once the journey home actually starts[8].

Precognition is knowledge of a future event that could not otherwise be anticipated. A typical example is suddenly thinking of someone only to have them call you or meet you a short time later. Another common example involves knowing who is calling you before you see any information about the call. A recent survey found that 80% of people claimed to have experienced one or other of these forms of precognition[9]. They especially occur between people who share a deep emotional bond. Try asking twins, or close siblings about their awareness of the others emotional states, even when they are far apart. Such experiences are so common that few of us stop to consider their implications. Anything this widespread, with such a high frequency and predictive accuracy can hardly be labeled a coincidence. If we take these events at face value, as genuine examples of direct or intuitive knowledge, they represent a major challenge to the mainstream understanding of both consciousness and reality. The following example is a fairly typical of my wife, Gulcan's intuitive work with a client in which she facilitates their use of the new class of energy psychology techniques.

"I was working with a client whose husband had died after a long and happy marriage. She had been unable to come to terms with his death and was overwhelmed by her grief. As we sat together a mental image came to me. It was of a man doing the washing-up at a kitchen sink, strong feelings of sadness and the message "I don't want you to do this". I asked the client what significance, if any, this image and message had for her. She immediately answered that throughout their long marriage her husband had always insisted on doing the washing up and never let her do it. Since his death she had kept herself continuously busy in the kitchen washing everything up and trying to connect with him. She understood that she had to give this up and that he would be happier if she got on with her life. The image and the message helped her to clear her grief using the energy psychology techniques."

What was so significant in this session was that a piece of obscure, highly personal but extremely precise information, the single piece of information necessary to trigger the healing process, occurred spontaneously to the healer at just the right time. Amongst experienced healers this happens quite frequently and forms an integral part of their expertise. Hidden in such apparently 'small' details are truths that should cause us to question our entire understanding of mind and our connections with the wider reality. Up to now we have dealt with spontaneous access to information with which we have an emotional connection, but not a physical one. We will now turn to deliberate attempts to access information with which we have no connection whatsoever.

Dowsing & Remote Viewing

My first exposure to dowsing came one day when I returned to a summer house we had rented to find a man 'purposefully' wandering around the garden. He had a small Yshaped stick in his hands. He walked around the front of the house, turned and then walked back around the side. He stopped and indicated a spot to the caretaker. I guessed they were busy with site management and left them to it. A week later on returning home I was confronted by a flat-bed truck with a crane mounted behind the cab and a mound of tubes on the back reversed up the driveway. At the side the house stood a 20 meter derrick. Tubes ran down and into the ground at the spot the man had indicated the week before. From the hole in the ground a great tide of mud oozed out and ran down the driveway and across the lawn. The man I had seen the week before had been a professional dowser. He had indicated a spot for drilling that would provide access to fresh water in what was otherwise a dry, barren landscape. The previous week he had announced that a good supply of fresh water would be found at a depth of 90 meters or so. The drilling crew hit fresh water at 110 meters.

Dowsing has traditionally been used to detect lost or hidden objects such as sources of water, oil or minerals. Detection is often performed using a pendulum or pointing rod. Such tools are not essential but they help the dowser to 'externalize' the answer to any question that they have asked. The dowsing response is intuitive, psycho-physical feedback that arises in answer to a specific question. Concerning his own approach the professional dowser, Hamish Miller, wrote, "It is all about tuning your mind. The aim is complete relaxation in body and thoughts but keeping one tiny part of your mind totally concentrated on the target"[10].

The dowsing response is probably one of the most familiar, and hence more acceptable, forms of remote sensing practice. It is one that just about everyone can learn and develop. There is, however, a big gap between the performance levels of interested amateurs and the professionals who earn their living from their ability. Is there any independent scientific evidence establishing the validity of this practice? In order to assess the effectiveness of its foreign aid contributions the German government undertook a 10 year, multi-nation study of the relative success rates of experienced dowsers in finding water as compared to conventional techniques. They found that the success rates of experienced dowsers were as high as 96% against an expected 30 – 50% using conventional techniques[11]. In addition, the dowsers were able to predict the depth and yield of a well to within 10 to 20% accuracy. This study was undertaken in areas of the world, such as sub-Saharan Africa, where water sources are especially deep and a deviation of just one meter either side could mean the difference between success and failure.

Dowsing is sometimes 'explained' as an interaction between the dowsing rod and subtle variations in the earth's electromagnetic fields resulting from sub-surface features such as water or minerals. In this case the dowsing instrument is thought of as acting like an 'aerial' that picks up and amplifies these subtle signals. There are two problems with this explanation. Firstly, it is possible to dowse an area without a dowsing instrument of any kind. Secondly, it is possible to dowse an area remotely. This can be done, for example, by dowsing a map. In this case the possible contribution of the area's electromagnetic fields hardly arises.

An acquaintance of ours, Ali Seydi Gultekin, a geological engineer as well as a professional dowser, is often called upon to provide the preliminary analysis of the water potential of plots of land situated on a different continent. He does this by dowsing the large aerial photographs of the plots that are sent to him. After selecting the most likely plots he flies in to carry out a more detailed study on the ground. Some of the people using his services are interested in investing in hotels in the desert around Las Vegas. They need to carefully evaluate the viability of underground water sources as a key element in managing the risks to the hundreds of millions dollars involved in such ventures. Their siting over ample, accessible sources of water is essential to their long-term viability. In his spare time he flies to Africa to work on a charitable basis locating and tapping supplies of underground water for remote villages.

Psi & the Limits of Knowledge

Most of us have experienced Psi at some time or other, even if it was just thinking of someone only to have them unexpectedly appear or call us. But at the core of the professional's expertise lays the ability to combine highly receptive modes of awareness with a focused intent towards locating some specific object or information. Their focused intent is sufficient to filter out everything that doesn't fit their search criteria. In other words, the Psi faculty operates as an open, intentionality directed search and locate mechanism with non-local capabilities. By 'non-local' I mean the ability to directly access information with which we have no physical connection. This may be because it is lost in the past, relates to the future, is hidden, unconscious or undisclosed. But if we have no physical connection with the source of the information, given the cases that we have looked at, we must have some other connection with it. Understanding the nature of this connection takes us to the very heart of the issue of what consciousness is. I suggest that Psi is a defining property of consciousness.

The anthropologist, Charles Laughlin, noted that many societies derive their knowledge from many different states of consciousness including Psi, intuition, dreams and visions. He calls these cultures 'polyphasic' and contrasts them with those societies whose largely 'monophasic' culture only credits experience had in 'normal' waking consciousness[12]. But as we saw, even in the most monophasic of the secular societies of modernity a large, and growing, segment of the population are willing to accept information derived through states of intuitive and empathic awareness. Outside of academia, mainstream science and media, the grassroots of western culture is, in many ways, profoundly polyphasic. The majority of people honor a variety of ways in which things can be known, though they tend to draw the line at information derived from the more extreme end of the spectrum, such as prophecy and divination.

Why is Psi so important?

The philosopher, Charles Taylor, sees the root of many modern ills, the characteristic sense of disengagement from and disenchantment with many aspects of life, as rooted in a loss of 'porosity' in relation to our selfhood; the openness, relatedness and 'enchantment' that comes through engaging empathically with life[13]. The ability to feel connected to all life forms is the key to our continued personal and spiritual development. It is also the key to our continued survival. Humanity is challenged to move beyond the unconscious demonization of other groups, peoples and cultures and its indifference to the destruction and pollution of the natural environment.

Around the world forces of globalization and industrialization are eroding bio and cultural diversity. We encounter the same brands, clothing, entertainment and food products wherever we go. Less commented on is the fact that this uniform consumer culture tends to undermine perceptual diversity – our natural ability to connect to reality using different states of awareness. By relating to others in an intuitive and empathic way, perceptual diversity implies a far more holistic engagement with reality. It is easy to see how such states play an important role in retaining harmony and balance within our own lives, within society and with the environment[14].

All three losses of diversity (bio, cultural, and perceptual) are closely related[15]. Once we open the door, so to speak, to other ways of knowing, when we accept that these states provide access to a broader, more connected understanding of reality, then our entire conception of the relationship between self and the environment has to change.

Holistic, intuitive and empathic ways of relating to reality are often thought of as sacrificing objectivity in favor of imagination or guesswork. In other words, information gained in these ways, even if it turns out to be true, can't qualify as knowledge. The classical definition of knowledge, one that has been around for at least 2,500 years, defines knowledge as 'justified, true, belief'. This formula has been passed down, unchanged, from Plato[16] to modern philosophy[17]. But because of the way in which our concept of 'justification' has evolved over the last 500 years or so, both intuitive and direct knowledge are thought to lack justification, that is, causal linkages that can be independently demonstrated to and reproduced by others. Intuitive and direct knowledge fail to meet these criteria for the simple reason that they are dependent upon each person's capacity for these special forms of perception. But as we saw in the German government study, the success rates of professional dowsers are consistently higher than those of conventional hydrologists. If these 'softer' forms of knowing produce results that are right more often than they are wrong, and a whole lot better than those available through conventional means, then we need to revisit our understanding of what constitutes knowledge. 'Knowledge', 'relevant facts' and 'truth' are as much determined by our cultural frame of reference as by what is 'out there'. The argument over the validity of Psi is as much a culture war as a debate about the evidence.

Developing our awareness in order to reliably access a much broader spectrum of reality has always required some degree of personal transformation. We find evidence of this amongst most of the world's remaining aboriginal peoples. We will examine one example, the Kalahari Kung 'healing dance'[18], later on. We also find evidence of the use of altered states as early as 40,000BCE as evidenced by cave paintings[19]. Throughout the IndoChinese, Asiatic and GrecoRoman worlds, philosophy involved numerous practical disciplines designed to affect personal transformation,

> "For the philosophical theme (how to have access to the truth) and the question of spirituality (what transformations in the being of the subject are necessary for access to the truth) were never separate." [20,21]

These ancient conceptions survived in Europe, though in an increasingly marginalized form, until at least the 16th Century when the emergence of modern science and the scientific method supplanted them. The benefit of this shift was that it cleared the way for the rapid advances in science and technology that we see continuing today. However, it also resulted in an enormous 'flattening' of our perspective on and insight into ourselves and a profound loss of connectedness with certain subtler, less obvious aspects of reality. One of the purposes of this book is to help to heal this breach and re-establish the older model of direct knowing alongside our modern conception.

Conclusions

From this brief review of some of the experiential and scientific evidence of psi we can draw a number of conclusions: First and foremost we need to remember that the challenge they present is not a challenge to science. It is, however, a challenge to the mainstream scientific understanding of consciousness and reality. The most extreme of these cases involves emotional reactions to or knowledge of future events. How can we sense or have knowledge of events that have yet to occur? In what possible sense could such events be said to 'exist'? And yet, as we have seen, numerous scientific experiments, and many first hand experiences, affirm that this is exactly what happens. If we accept the validity of these experiences then surely we must find ourselves in conflict with both commonsense and scientific conceptions of time?

The disparity between the understanding of consciousness and reality revealed by experiences of Psi and our day to day experience is so great that it should give us pause for thought. Is there something missing in mainstream understanding? Our present moment of awareness is always a momentary 'snapshot'. It is the self's unique 'point of view'. But if, as the evidence suggests, our awareness can be spatially and temporally displaced or refocused to access different times and places or to intercept other's thoughts, feelings and memories, then we surely need a different model of consciousness and its relationship with reality. Perhaps by examining the most extreme, rare and subtle manifestations of awareness we can begin to discern the outlines of what this model might look like?

From an experiential point of view we can think of intuitive perception as arising from a movement or shift of our awareness within the broader spectrum of consciousness – whose composition and boundaries we have yet to understand. This movement is experienced as a progressive broadening of our awareness and a corresponding shrinking of our sense of a discrete, biographically constructed self. The progressive broadening of our awareness moves through a spectrum of defocalized states. We can categorize these states in a number of ways, the following sequence represents just one way of doing so. The sequence runs from present moment awareness through instinctive, intuitive, empathic, and psychic modes. This scale is experienced by most of us, though states above the level of 'empathic' become progressively rarer.

With a broadening of our awareness, our orientation towards the here and now, our connectedness to mundane reality and sense of selfhood, begin to dissolve. With this, we begin to gain access non-local information – information from beyond the boundaries of our immediate senses. As we saw, this information may relate to events, people or objects with which we have no physical connection.

Beyond these modes, certain psychic modes of awareness become accessible. Amongst very gifted healers, many of whom can access this level of awareness, information about the energy body, the deep emotional causes of ill health and misfortune and the effects of past lives can become transparent. Progressing beyond these psychic modes of awareness we begin to access the states of unitive and non-dual awareness characteristic of the world's mystical traditions. Our awareness may come to feel 'oceanic'. And like any fathomless space it arouses both our curiosity – and our fear. For the limitless, like the formless, threatens to engulf our identity entirely.

The capacity to experience these states is a natural one, albeit one that is innately stronger in some people. It is therefore a capability that can be further trained and developed. We have seen that under suitable conditions it provides a path to direct knowledge and understanding. In the next chapter we will see how these states of knowing access 'deep memory', the remembrance that runs back through our biographical time line to include past lives and ancestral memories that directly affect our health and well-being.

Diagram II: Field-like Structure of Defocalized Awareness

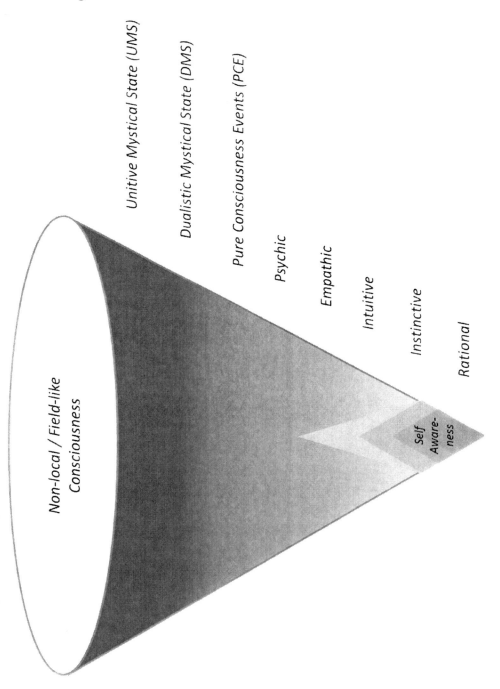

Notes

1. Haraldsson, E. & Hootkouper, JM. 'Psychic Experience in the Multinational Human Values Study: Who Reports Them?' Journal of the American Society for Psychical Research, Volume 85, April 1991, 145-165

2. Levin, JS. 'Age Differences in Mystical Experience' The Gerontologist, 1993, Volume: 33(4): 507-513

3. Bem, DJ. 'Feeling the Future: Experimental Evidence for Anomalous Retroactive Influences on Cognition and Affect' Journal of Personality and Social Psychology, March 2011, Volume 100(3), 407-425

4. Radin, D. (1997) 'Unconscious Perception of Future Emotions: An Experiment in Presentiment' Journal of Scientific Exploration, Vol. 11, No. 2, pp. 163-180, 1997

5. Bierman, DJ. & Radin, DI., (1997) 'Anomalous anticipatory response on randomized future conditions' Perceptual and Motor Skills, 84, 689-690

6. Spottiswoode, P. & May, E., (2003) 'Skin Conductance Prestimulus Response: Analyses, Artifacts and a Pilot Study' Journal of Scientific Exploration, Vol. 17, No. 4, pp. 617-641.

7. Tressoldi, PE., Martinelli, M., Massaccesi, S., & Sartori, L., (2005) 'Heart Rate Differences between Targets and Non-targets in Intuitive Tasks' Human Physiology, Vol. 31, No. 6, 2005, pp. 646–650

8. Sheldrake, R. 'A Dog That Seems To Know When His Owner is Coming Home: Videotaped Experiments and Observations' Journal of Scientific Exploration (2000) 14, 233-255

9. Breen, R. 'The Nature Incidence and Impact of Paranormal Experiences' Monash University Survey, 2008

10. Miller, H. (2002) Dowsing: a Journey Beyond Our Senses

11. Betz, H-D. 'Unconventional Water Detection: Field Test of

the *Dowsing Technique in Dry Zones' Journal of Scientific Exploration, 1995, Vol. 9, No. I, pp. 1-43*

12. Laughlin, C. *'Consciousness in Biogenetic Structural Theory' Anthropology of Consciousness, 1992, 3(1-2):17-22.*

13. Taylor, C. *(2007) A Secular Age*

14. Lumpkin, TW. *'Perceptual Diversity and its Implications for Development—Based on Research among Traditional Healers and upon Community Use of Traditional Medicine in Namibia, March 1996.' PhD Thesis*

15. Lumpkin, TW. *'Perceptual Diversity: Is Polyphasic Consciousness Necessary for Global Survival?' Anthropology of Consciousness, Vol. 12, No. 1, March/June 2001*

16. Plato *Theaetetus 201b-d*

17. Ayer, AJ. *(1956) The Problem of Knowledge*

18. Katz, R. 1982. *Boiling Energy. Community Healing Among the Kalahari Kung*

19. Lewis-Williams, DJ. *(2002) The Mind In The Cave: Consciousness and the Origins of Art*

20. Foucault, M. *(2005) The Hermeneutics of the Subject: Lectures at the College de France 1981-82 p.17*

21. Hadot, P. *(1995) Philosophy as a Way of Life: spiritual exercises from Socrates to Foucault*

Chapter 3

Healing issues within our time-line

When do 'we' begin?

John was a successful, aspiring manager with a large multinational corporation. His natural grace, good manners and generosity marked him as someone most people would like to know. But appearances can belie the suffering that overshadows many people's inner lives. John came to me suffering from deep seated, persistent feelings of loneliness. Feelings that haunted him no matter where he was or whose company he was in. He wanted to see whether rebirthing breathwork would help him. Rebirthing Breathwork is a powerful technique that utilizes a form of connected breathing, called 'circular breathing', to rapidly increase the level of our inner energy. The increased energy tends to activate any deepseated personal issues that lay beneath the surface of our conscious awareness. During his third session John suddenly started moving violently. From a laying position he jerked up and down from the waist and from side to side, as though trying to escape from some tight confinement. Finally his movements subsided. He experienced cold, darkness, and feelings of abandonment and loneliness. Suddenly he sat up and announced "It's done!" He felt clear and focused. Something had clearly integrated at a very deep level. I later learned that when still in his mother's womb, his mother's waters had broken and she had been unable to get to a hospital for many hours. Unable to commence the birth process the baby experienced the womb as a dark, cold, lonely place. It was this experience that had haunted him throughout his life and which had now re-surfaced and been integrated during the rebirthing session. The powerful movements back and forth re-enacted those of the baby trying to get free of the womb before exhaustion, and a sense of overwhelming loneliness, overcame it. In the following weeks, John searched carefully for any traces of his former deep-seated loneliness but of the feelings that had haunted him all of his life, not a trace remained.

We normally think of the source of emotional disturbances as occurring in childhood. But some troubles appear to have much deeper roots. As we saw in John's case, significant life issues can be connected to the nature of our birth process. Problems at this stage routinely surface, and are resolved, during Rebirthing Breathwork. But as we will see, some issues have their origins far earlier. The following cases are drawn from Gulcan's case files.

"Anne was a well educated professional in her 40s who was troubled by her continuing codependency on her mother. Despite the fact that she had lived independently abroad for many years, educating herself and establishing a career, she still felt impelled to return to her home country in order to be closer to her mother. At the same time she felt dislike for her and a feeling that her mother had never loved her. She said, "One part of me wants so much to stay with her and the other part of me has to leave her. I'm so divided. I need my mother's love, but somehow I'm very angry with her". Applying a meridian therapy technique (in this case Emotional Freedom Techniques or EFT) she remembered a moment when she was silently screaming, "Please let me live! I promise I will never be a burden for you".

Through the healing process it became clear that her mother had, in the early months of pregnancy, made a decision to have an abortion. She was only stopped from going through with it because her husband had insisted that he wanted her to have the baby. The client had reported feeling a great fear that "The opportunity for life" would be lost if her mother went through with the abortion. It was a contract made while she was still in her mother's womb. In her effort to fulfill her side of the bargain "Never to be a burden" if she was allowed to live, as soon as she was able, she had felt impelled to take responsibility for every aspect of her life so as not to have to depend upon her mother for anything."

The mainstream medical conception of consciousness is that it is a by-product of neurological development in the third trimester, that is, somewhere between the seventh and ninth months of pregnancy. This is clearly mistaken and leads to the denial of awareness to a broad spectrum of life. The case strongly suggests that all sentient life has awareness, can sense danger and feel threatened, irrespective of where they are in their lifecycle. These facts have major ethical implications. Stanislav Grof, a psychiatrist and one of the founders of the transpersonal movement in psychology, noted,

"The idea that a functioning consciousness could exist in a fetus was in conflict with everything he had, been taught in medical school...that he could be aware of subtle nuances between himself and his mother ... astonished him"[1]

One more of Gulcan's cases will help to establish this point. "A psychotherapist came to me for help with a deep seated snake phobia. The phobia was so acute that any snake-like shape – a spiraling bamboo in the corner and even a road winding into the distance – triggered an extremely fearful reaction. Using a meridian therapy technique (in this case Tapas Acupressure Technique or TAT) it became evident that the client had never actually seen a snake, let alone had a traumatic experience of one. It turned out that when still in his mother's womb, his mother had encountered a large snake in the kitchen. People in the house were screaming, "Look how it curves!", "Look how fast it is!" Caught up in these reactions, the mother's fear was transferred to the fetus creating a phobia that, in the mature person, existed with no corresponding experience."

Cases like this serve to highlight the point that a person's recoverable history reaches back beyond the point of birth. How far that may be, and to what extent their 'memories' are their 'own', is the object of our inquiry.

"If I accept that the patterns are mother's emotional-mental patterns then what I am experiencing during some regression therapies are not actually my own experiences – because I am not wholly me yet – but are my mother's pre-birth and labour feeling patterns"[2].

The power of techniques like Rebirthing breathwork, used in John's case, arise from the connection between our breath, our 'inner energy' and the quality of our awareness. This connectivity has been recognized and utilized by shaman, yogis and mystics for thousands of years. As the holistic physician, Deepak Chopra, observed, "Breath is the junction point between mind, body and spirit". The form of breathing used in these forms of breathwork is called 'circular breathing'. It consists in connecting the inhale and exhale in one smooth circuit whilst pulling the inhale and completely relaxing the exhale, so that it takes care of itself. Circular breathing is always preceded by relaxation exercises and accompanied by complete muscular relaxation. It should never be attempted without experienced supervision or training since things can get out of hand very rapidly. Its main effect is to very rapidly increase the level of our 'inner energy'. This has two effects: firstly, it activates and facilitates the integration of deep seated emotional issues; secondly, it facilitates the onset of a greatly expanded depth and quality of awareness. From this it will be evident that 'inner energy' is fundamental to understanding consciousness, healing and transformation. In fact, this is exactly what ancient traditions affirm. Because of the points raised by these case histories we need to explore the concept of 'inner energy' and understand its connection to consciousness in more detail.

Inner Energy

Inner energy is also called 'vital energy' or 'subtle energy'. More commonly it is known as Qi (pronounced 'chi') in Eastern healing, yogic and martial disciplines. In Eastern tradition Qi is always accompanied by consciousness or Li. Qi and Li are thought of as being inseparable. A traditional Eastern metaphor for this relationship is that of the blind horse and the lame rider. The blind horse (representing Qi) has the power to move lacks direction or agency. Conversely the lame rider (representing consciousness or Li) has vision (a sense of direction or agency) but lacks the ability to move. In other words, consciousness and energy are intimately intertwined; you cannot have one without the other. This alternative model of consciousness sees it as a universal field rather than the byproduct, or epiphenomena, of neural activity. We need to consider which of these models best explains the cases of healing and transformation recorded throughout this book.

A store of innate Qi energy exists in each sentient being. This energy can be enhanced by energy absorbed from the earth, the air we breathe and the food we eat. In John's case breathing and relaxation were sufficient to drive his level of Qi energy up to such a level that it both surfaced and facilitated the integration of the deep seated emotional blockage related to his traumatic birth experience.

Less well known is the fact that Qi energy can also be 'drawn down' in a form known as 'universal energy'. This form of energy provides the healing energy used in the many forms of hands-on healing that have been practiced from time immemorial. In recent years hands-on healing has become very popular. One tradition that has fuelled this popularity is the once esoteric Japanese practice of Reiki (more specifically it is called Usui Reiki, after its founder Mikao Usui). This form of the hands-on healing is easy to acquire, since it only requires a short 'initiation' process to activate it, and is highly effective. It can prove especially effective in situations that conventional medicine is unable to address, as Gulcan's mother demonstrated.

"One day I noticed that my 75 year old mother had a few of bruises on her arms and legs. Since she had not had any accidents, I suspected that it could be due to internal bleeding. When she visited the doctor he confirmed that this was the problem. His diagnosis was that the spleen was failing to let go of the platelets that thicken the blood and allow it to clot (Thrombocytopenia). The bone marrow was producing blood cells but the spleen would not release them into the bloodstream. Normally the number of platelets should be between 200,000 and 450,000 per microliter of blood. My mother's count was just 8,000. If she had cut herself, the blood would not have been able to clot and would not stop flowing. At first the doctor tried Cortisone. The platelet count increased to 160,000 but then fell back down to 30,000 by the end of the treatment. This was still far too low. She was told to wait since nothing more could be done at this stage. The spleen could not be removed since the thin blood would make any operation problematic, and in any case they did not know whether this procedure would work. At this stage I told my mother to set her mind to get well and to start using her first degree Reiki on herself. She accepted this advice and started to systematically apply Reiki to her spleen every day for a few hours. The monthly platelet counts started to increase. First, they went up to 60,000, then to 145,000, and then up again to 195,000. When they reached 195,000 her doctor, the head of the Hematology department at the university hospital, became curious. He asked her if she was undergoing some other treatment. She told him about Usui Reiki, about which he showed a lot of interest, and said, "Whatever you're doing, please continue, it's good for you!" After 4-5 months of systematic, daily self-treatment she was completely and permanently healed. A few years later, at a conference at which I was one of the speakers I told this story and thanked the doctor, mentioning his name because he had been so open-minded and supportive. Somebody in the audience stood up and said "He is also practicing Reiki now".

Needless to say, despite the existence of scientific research about hands-on healing, neither Reiki nor any other form of hands-on healing is recognized by mainstream Western culture or medical practice[3]. In fact, skeptics routinely dismiss the idea as 'vitalism', the superstitious attribution of supernatural agency to inanimate matter. In doing so, Western science has overlooked the one essential concept that facilitates an understanding of the nature and scope of consciousness. Whilst mainstream Western science and culture continue to be oblivious to the existence of these energy fields, this is not true for the rest of the world. Research into the nature of Qi energy continues to be undertaken in countries, such as China[4] and Japan[5], where the concept forms an integral part of their cultural traditions and practices.

Qi energy flows through the body and to the major organs via a set of channels, called meridians. The system of meridians provides the basis for a whole range of healing modalities of which perhaps the best known is the ancient practice of acupuncture. Acupuncture is commonly thought of as an extremely ancient Chinese practice[6]. But as the following account shows, this may be an oversimplification.

In 1991 the frozen body of a man was found encased in the ice, high on the mountains bordering Italy and Austria. Carbon dating revealed it to be over 5,000 years old. The body had been well preserved because of the cold, dry conditions that had endured there for millennia. Medical examination determined that the man had suffered from a number of health problems, specifically arthritis of the lumbar spine and a digestive disorder. But the most remarkable finding was that the body had some 15 groups of simple tattoos on it, none of which appeared to have any ritual or ornamental significance. Instead, 80% of the 58 tattoos corresponded exactly with the points used by modern acupuncturists to treat the two conditions that the man had been diagnosed as suffering from[7]. An expert opinion on the placement of the tattoos was sought from one of the main Chinese colleges of traditional medicine. Their specialists concluded that two thirds of the tattoos had been placed on the primary location used to treat back pain and that the remainder were located on or around points used to treat problems associated with digestion[8]. Apparently early European healers shared the same understanding of the energy-body and how to work with it to heal and relieve pain as contemporary acupuncturists. This remarkable convergence of diagnosis and practice in different cultures separated by millennia and on different sides of the planet suggests that the same underlying reality is being perceived, understood and managed to alleviate suffering and promote healing.

More recently experimentation with the relationship between the major meridians and physical and emotional problems has led to the development of a whole range of new and highly effective meridian therapies. Chief amongst these are Gary Craig's 'Emotional Freedom Technique' (EFT) and Tapas Fleming's 'Tapas Acupressure Technique' (TAT). The fact that these easy to learn and apply techniques are capable of eliminating conditions that defy conventional medicine supports the underlying model of energy, consciousness and healing on which they are based.

The Energy-body & Negative Emotions

"At a company meeting I was invited to give a talk on health & happiness to the management team. In order to demonstrate the power of the new energy psychology techniques to empower more effective self-management I asked the audience of 100 or so managers whether anyone had a problem that they would like to resolve. A woman put her hand up. Her problem was an acute fear of public speaking. Because her fear was so intense she could not speak up and I had to go to her. She was shaking when I joined her in the audience. I started to tap on the woman's meridian points using the standard Emotional Freedom Techniques (EFT) protocol and asked everyone else in the audience to 'tap along' with the lady intending that they were her. At this point they had received no information or training about the technique. Nevertheless, after just two rounds of tapping the woman's fear was entirely eliminated and she was able to come to the front of the room and comfortably address the entire audience."

Cases like this are common amongst the people who work professionally with these techniques. To the 'outsider' they appear to be incredible, if not impossible. The gap between these two lived realities, between that of the professional energy healer and most other people is large. The question that we wanted to address was how the energy-body and negative emotions are related to physical illness and mental disorder. In order to answer this we need to have a view about what a 'negative emotion' is. For sure, it is a tendency to feel sad, fearful or angry, to react in certain ways and to be subject to certain recurring thoughts or memories. In meridian therapy terms a negative emotion is, at root, a restriction to the free flow of lifeenergy. Merely tapping the meridians is sufficient to complete release even the deepest emotional pain, trauma and anxiety. Our potential to re-shape our lives, and to help others, is far more dynamic than many of us imagine. It is more dynamic than many of us can even begin to imagine. Fortunately we are now beginning to see the first serious studies of the effectiveness of these new techniques.

In the case of the new meridian therapies, the experiential and experimental evidence is clear: maintaining a clear and present focus on a specific negative emotion whilst tapping or otherwise stimulating the major meridians results in its complete and permanent release. When that emotion is underpinning a physical problem (most back pain for example) the removal of the underlying emotion will cause the physical problem to disappear. The same procedure can mitigate, if not remove, a large percentage of purely physical aches and pains directly. Over the last 20 years the validity of this process has been proven countless times with every form of negative emotion – fear, sadness, anger – and even with the most severe and intractable of anxiety disorders such as Post-Traumatic Stress Disorder (PTSD)[9,10]. This was demonstrated as long ago as the 1980s when Gary Craig worked with veterans of the Vietnam War, some of whom had suffered from PTSD for over 20 years. Gary used a simple, easy to use meridian therapy that he had developed from an earlier technique called Thought Field Therapy. Gary's streamlined version is called Emotional Freedom Techniques (EFT)[11]. EFT involves remaining focused upon a specific mental, emotional or physical discomfort whilst tapping a small number of the key energy meridians. As the tapping progresses the level of discomfort starts to fall until it is entirely eliminated. Success rates with this technique, especially when it is facilitated by an experienced user, are around 90%.

A recent randomized study of veterans suffering from PTSD saw 70% of the EFT group score PTSDnegative after just 3 sessions and 87% score PTSDnegative after just 6 sessions[12]. In the context of such an otherwise intractable problem as PTSD, these scores are little short of miraculous and far beyond anything achievable through conventional approaches. And yet despite overwhelming evidence for its effectiveness, the technique has been almost completely ignored by mainstream media, biology, medicine and psychotherapy. It simply does not conform to mainstream Western biomedical models of reality. It is also free and therefore of little interest to profit driven Western medicine. Anyone can watch the abundance of 'how to' videos through online media and download a manual for free. It is easy to learn and fun to apply, highly effective, natural and with no side effects.

The importance of these techniques, apart from their immense value in empowering people to overcome a vast range of mental, emotional and physical conditions, is that they clearly illustrate the interdependence of our mental, physical and emotional health and well-being with our energy system – a system that is entirely unrecognized by western biological and medical science.

There is, however, a further reason for dwelling on these techniques. They have something of fundamental importance to teach us about the nature of reality and consciousness. Not only does tapping the meridians work to alleviate or eliminate all kinds of health issues, imagining that you are tapping them also works not quite as well, admittedly, but it does work! And 'surrogate' tapping, imagining that you are someone else and tapping yourself on their behalf, also works, even if the person is on the other side of the planet. This is, of course, a major challenge to conventional thinking and to mainstream science. Nevertheless, it is a part of the daily experience of energy healers worldwide. Let's briefly recount another of Gulcan's cases.

"I received a call from a distraught woman whose young daughter had just been diagnosed with deafness. She was very upset about it and afraid that the condition could worsen. She had no knowledge of the meridian therapies that she might use to help herself. I asked for permission to act as a surrogate for her. She was happy to give this. I then applied the standard remote meridian therapy protocol to myself as though I was the client. Within a couple of minutes the woman's upset had completely disappeared, even though she was hundreds of miles away."

From the point of view of consensual reality such claims are beyond anything that most people can possibly imagine, let alone accept. Nevertheless, that is how reality and consciousness are structured. Our approach is neither philosophical nor speculative. It is based upon thousands of cases that attest to the truth of these statements. I believe that our whole view about the nature of reality and its relationship to consciousness needs an upgrade to bring it into line with 21st century experience. While we think of consciousness as the shifting domain of our own local awareness, in fact it behaves more as though it was a part of a much larger, shared whole in which we all partake and which has distinctive 'field-like' properties. This is not a theoretical supposition. It is simply the best way of describing the actual experience of working with these techniques.

The Mind-Body Connection

The connection between the energy-body and our quality of awareness is a direct one. Is it also a two way connection? Mindfulness is a form of meditative practice that consists in maintaining a state of present moment, non-judgmental awareness. Mindfulness is easy to describe but experience shows that, for most people at least, it is difficult to maintain for any length of time. Like riding a bike, mindfulness is a practical skill that is easy to learn but only mastered through regular practice. Recent research on the effects of mindfulness has demonstrated greatly reduced levels of stress and increased immune system functioning[13]. More significantly, it has demonstrated that although mindfulness meditation might look like 'just doing nothing' the areas of the brain that are activated in clinically depressed and anxious people become much less so and there is increased activation in the areas associated with happiness and contentment. This shift in neural activity is also associated with the growth (neurogenesis) and development (neuroplasticity) of the neural networks that sustain such positive states[14]. People who practice mindfulness are less deeply impacted by negative events and recover far more quickly when they do occur. In other words, health, happiness and contentment are outcomes of the cultivation of quietude and acceptance, and these are practical skills that can be refined and developed through practice.

Recent medical research has established the value of mindfulness as an adjunct treatment for a whole range of illnesses. The research underlying these findings is consistent with that emerging from the rapidly growing discipline of Positive Psychology. Positive Psychology is the study of happiness and positivity and their effects on human health and wellbeing. Barbara Fredrickson, a leading researcher, has summarized the benefits of positive emotions as[15]:

- Widening the scope of people's attention, broadening their behavioral repertoires and increasing intuition and creativity.
- Boosting immune function, so that people are less prone to illness, and hastening their recovery if they do become sick.
- Increasing resilience to adversity and promoting happiness and psychological growth.
- Predicting how long people live.

In other words, positivity – what we do with our minds, how we choose to think and deploy our awareness from moment to moment – has powerful effects on just about every area of life.

When do 'we' end?

An acquaintance of ours, Stephen, was a professional sportsman. He provided us with the following account of an experience that ended his professional career.

"I was having my Summer holiday with friends. We drank a lot at a club and I refused to drive us back to the hotel. But my friend said that he felt sick and begged me to drive. I can only remember that an instant after we entered the main road we had a crash. I remember feeling totally free and completely at peace for the first time in my life as I gazed out across the beautiful landscape. Suddenly I felt a powerful 'pull' as though I was being removed from the scene of the accident. I found myself looking down on the accident. I saw the wrecked car, bodies lying on the road and people covering them. I recognized one of the bodies as my own. I remember thinking that my time had not come yet and that I wanted to return and live the rest of my life; and with that, in a flash, I was back 'inside' my body which was racked with tremendous pain."

In this accident Stephen lost his friends and a promising career. After several operations involving the insertion of steel plates, it still took him two years to achieve some degree of physical recovery. Near Death Experiences (NDE), such as this account provided by a friend of ours, occur when a person experiences clinical death (their heart stops) and after being resuscitated they recall significant events related to their death. Research has shown that between one and two thirds of people who have died and been resuscitated have had a near death experience. In the case of children this figure is even higher. Some of the experiences that people typically cite include: experiencing positive emotions, being aware of having died, meeting with deceased persons, moving through a tunnel, visiting a celestial landscape, having an out of body experience, communicating with light, observing colors and experiencing a 'life review'. NDE may also include additional elements such as: being greeted by 'higher beings', becoming aware of or being told that it is not their time to die and that they need to return, the ability to recount details about the situation around them after they have died that they could not have known about. Finally, many people who have these experiences report finding a renewed sense of purpose in life, acknowledging the reality of a spiritual dimension to existence and overcoming their fear of death. Many people view these phenomena as hallucinations. But this fails to account for those situations in which detailed information about events that took place around them after they have died, are recalled. Out of body experiences accompany NDE in around one quarter of cases. There are ample first-hand accounts of people witnessing what was taking place around them after they had died. Another acquaintance had the following, life-changing experience. Another acquaintance of ours, Mark, a senior management consultant who had made light of our energy work, provided us with the following account.

"After suffering a heart attack I was engulfed in a great light and felt a great sense of peace and lightness. I found myself looking down on a still figure on a bed being rushed through a hospital and then undergoing a medical procedure. I watched as one of the nurses knocked over a tray of instruments that fell and scattered across the floor. A doctor was working on a body. I suddenly recognized it as mine! He applied a defibrillator to my chest. I suddenly felt a big pain followed by intense tingling in my chest area. I also felt very heavy as I was suddenly encumbered with my body once more. A day or so later, I mentioned the incident of the dropped instruments to the doctor who was surprised that I knew about it. After all, I was dead at the time."

After his experience Mark went on to become a Reiki teacher. On one occasion he helped a man who had been paralyzed from the neck down to regain movement in his arms by using Reiki for distance healing.

Such accounts suggest a number of important factors relating to the nature of consciousness and reality. Firstly, that we are able to separate our awareness from our bodies. Secondly, in this state we can access information that would not, otherwise, be accessible to us. Thirdly, in a large number of cases, death leaves our awareness intact, at least for some period of time. If consciousness were just a by-product of neural activity this would not be possible. The fact that accounts like this are reported in at least a third of NDE demonstrates the continuity of awareness after death and the separability of our awareness from our bodies.

In the next chapter we will continue to extend our exploration of the boundaries of consciousness and selfhood by looking at cases in which the origins of a disturbance or trauma emerges from beyond the limits of biographical history.

Notes

1. Grof, S. (1992) *The Holotropic Mind: The Three Levels of Human Consciousness & How They Shape Our Lives p.34*

2. Jon, RG & Troya, GN 'Rebirthing or Rebreathing : A Recapitualation' *The Healing Breath Volume 2 Number 3 September 2000 p.*

3. Seto, A. et al 'Detection of extraordinary large bio-magnetic field strength from human hand during external Qi emission' *Acupuncture & Electrotherapeutics Research. 1992; Volume 17, No. 2:75-94.*

4. Hui Lin 'Overview of the Status of Chinese Chi Research', *International Yan Xin Qigong Association.*

5. Kokubo, H. 'Concept of "Qi" or "Ki" in Japanese Qigong Research' *Proceedings of the 44th Annual Convention of the Parapsychological Association pp.147-154, 2001, New York*

6. Ma, Kan-Wen 'The Roots & Development of Chinese Acupuncture' *Acupuncture in Medicine 1992 Volume 10 Supplement*

7. Dorfer, L. et al 'A medical report from the stone age?' *The Lancet, 1999; 354: 1023–25*

8. 'Expert opinion concerning the tattoos on the Tyrolean iceman' *Beijing, Shanghai and Nanking Colleges of Traditional Chinese Medicine*

9. Church, D. Geronilla, L. & Dinter, I. 'Psychological Symptom Change in Veterans after Six Sessions of Emotional Freedom Techniques (EFT): An Observational Study' *The International Journal of Healing & Caring, Volume 9, Number 1, December 2009*

10. Church, D. 'The Treatment of Combat Trauma in Veterans Using EFT: A Pilot Protocol' *Traumatology, March 2010, Vol.16 No.1 55-65*

11. *It was a greatly simplified version of a technique developed by Dr.Roger Callahan called Thought Field Therapy*

12. *Church, D. et al. (2013) Psychological Trauma Symptom Improvement in Veterans Using Emotional Freedom Techniques: A Randomized Controlled Trial. The Journal of Nervous & Mental Disease. 201(2):153-160, February 2013.*

13. *Davidson, RJ., Kabat-Zinn, J. et al. 'Alterations in Brain and Immune Function Produced by Mindfulness Meditation'. Psychosomatic Medicine 65:564–570 (2003)*

14. *Davidson, RJ. & Lutz, Antoine 'Buddha's Brain: Neuroplasticity and Meditation' IEEE Signal Processing Magazine [174] January 2008*

15. *Fredrickson, B 'The Broaden & Build Theory of Positive Emotions' Philosophical Transactions of the Royal Society, August 2004, 359, 1367–1377*

Chapter 4

Healing issues beyond our time-line

Merged Identities

The cases that we have dealt with up to now remain within the range of most people's world view. What helps to keep them within the bounds of the familiar is that all of these cases refer to events within the subject's biographical time line. We are reassured by the continuity of the subject's physical presence. No matter how outlandish these cases appear to be, they do not necessitate a fundamental re-adjustment or re-set to most people's underlying beliefs. There is, however, a class of cases, regularly encountered in the context of energy healing, for which this reassuring continuity is absent. These cases provide a much more profound challenge to conventional notions of self-hood, consciousness and reality. We will now illustrate how the healing of deep personal issues can reveal deep seated causes in events that preceded the subject's conception. To make these points we will once more borrow from Gulcan's case files.

"Janet, is an art teacher, in her early thirties, with dark beautiful eyes and a hesitant voice. She came to me complaining that the meridian therapy that she had learned did not work for her. She needed help since she had felt depressed all her life, though she had not suffered any major traumas that would account for this. She had been to a number of psychotherapists, had used various anti-depressants off and on and tried a variety of complementary therapies. Nothing had worked for her. First of all I tested her using kinesiology, a technique for testing people's unconscious beliefs, but I could not even get a positive response to her name. Next I had her perform an exercise to re-balance her energy. This involved having the client touch their right elbow to their left knee and left elbow to their right knee a number of times. I then tested her once more using kinesiology and she now responded strongly to her name. Testing with kinesiology showed that she did not accept any kind of healing. To address her resistance we started clearing the issues around not deserving to live and not accepting love, help or healing. All of a sudden, she was in tears and said "I don't want to live". When I checked with her it emerged that she had felt suicidal and ten years before had actually attempted suicide. The reason for this was a deep seated feeling of guilt that she had felt all her life but for no apparent reason. I now checked whether she had a sibling who had died before her, whether from a miscarriage, abortion or early death. Janet replied, "Yes" – her mother had had a miscarriage at four months – "What's that got to do with it?" to which I replied "We'll see if it has anything to do with it". We next started clearing issues around "Two years before my birth, my sibling died". After a while it came to her that "My sibling died and I took their right to live". She felt that this was in some way her fault. "It feels like I'm responsible for their death," she said. She experienced a deep sense of guilt and pain because of this. We then worked to clear each of these negative feelings. Towards the end of the treatment, she took a deep breath and smiled. She felt light; her guilt and pain had gone and she felt herself to be innocent and free. In one session, we had cleared her resistance to meridian therapies, resistance to healing and ultimately, resistance to life itself. The reason for her depression was also cleared. Janet's voice had changed. She said loudly, "It worked! This is so liberating. Guilt? What a silly idea! Why on earth have I felt this guilt?".

Although everyone's case is unique, variations on this particular scenario have recurred many times. The loss of a sibling before one is born can lead to a deep and unconscious guilt, quite literally, 'survivor's guilt'. Children born after the death of a sibling may feel burdened by a sense of responsibility for the life of the dead child - even when they are completely unaware of the fact that such a fetus or child had existed. This is, of course, completely incredible to anyone 'stuck' in the emergentist view of consciousness that sees each person isolated within their own biographical history. Let's take one more of Gulcan's cases to emphasize the point.

"A young man came to me suffering with depression and an eating problem. He had been in psychotherapy but felt that 'it was going nowhere' and discontinued it. I learned from his mother that she had lost her first son. He had died aged three, six years before my client was born. When I mentioned this to him he stated that he had no particular feelings about it. But when we started to work with the deeper levels of consciousness using Tapas Acupressure Technique (TAT) he had an emotional breakthrough. He burst out crying, saying that he felt so sorry and so guilty, that he had no right to be alive when his brother should have lived. This powerful upsurge of feelings came as a complete surprise to him, since he had no prior feelings concerning the loss of this brother long before he was born. We worked through these negative feelings eliminating them one by one. At the end of the session he stated that a huge weight had been lifted off him. It was as if he had 'taken over' a load of sorrow on behalf of his brother."

These cases clearly demonstrate that we are unconsciously connected in a-temporal ways to family and ancestral currents of feeling that invisibly influence our health and happiness, sometimes in very negative ways. But as these cases illustrate, it is possible to isolate and eliminate these influences and free ourselves from their effects. None of these cases could be treated by conventional psychotherapy for the simple reason that there was no obvious trauma or upset underpinning the depression that the people suffered from. All of these cases are 'impossible' according to the mainstream understanding that limits consciousness to a person's biographical history. And it is just for this reason that these cases are so important. They demonstrate that our conventional understanding of consciousness is fundamentally mistaken. One more case along these lines also involves the loss of a sibling before a person's birth and its lingering effects on them. But in this case the sibling had a different, and rather special, relationship with the subject, as Gulcan explains,

"Helen was young, sharply dressed, good looking, successful corporate media director. After a 15 year relationship she finally married the man. 3 years later, even though there were no problems in the relationship, she divorced him. A year and a half later she was in another happy relationship. After just 2 years, she left him as well. Helen came to me complaining that she wasn't happy, she felt depressed and that each time she found happiness she couldn't help sabotaging it. In her youth she had seen many happy, long term relationships in her family. She was also afraid of being happy, fearing that it would go wrong.

She had had a sibling who had died 2 years before she was born. When I asked her about him she said, "I can't talk about him ... I don't even want to hear his name and I don't want to deal with that". After I had explained to her that the dead sibling may be affecting her in terms of her depression, tension and her sabotaging of her relationships she agreed to deal with her feelings about him. Just talking about the sibling made her cry. Whilst doing TAT she visualized the boy and talked to him saying, "You died before me and I'm very sorry for that. I accept you as my brother and into the family. I now let you go to the light." At this she cried even more. In her mind she 'heard' him answer, "I had to go so that you could come". This confused both of us. Normally in these situations the sibling will answer to the effect that "It wasn't your fault" and then just go. This invariably 'liberates' the person from the burden of negative feelings that they have been carrying. But because this response was so different I decided to use kinesiology (muscle testing) to try to understand what had happened by asking questions of the unconscious field of her experience.

To the statement, "My sibling died before me, it was his life, I shouldn't have taken it" she tested weak and experienced no feelings of guilt. To the statement, "I was him and I died as a child" she tested very strong and felt the full force of its truth throughout her body. This would be consistent with other pastlife death traumas, though in this case she had been her own sibling. We then went on to clear the emotional issues related to her sense of loneliness, sorrow and missing her mother and father. She next used the energy psychology protocol to clear associated feelings using the statements, "In that life I had to die early. I can now leave that life behind. I am so glad that I was able to come to the same, and correct, family". With this the trauma was fully released, "I can be happy now". After this she said that she had never felt better in all of her life. In the subsequent days everyone who knew her commented on her positivity and the change that had come over her. One week later she said that her life had changed. She felt a great happiness and much more 'connected'.

She called her mother to learn how the boy had died. It was from a respiratory illness and he had had to be quarantined and could have no contact with his father and mother before he died. This accounts for the loneliness that she had suffered from."

Modern culture and its system of healthcare remain hobbled by a refusal to recognize the field-like nature of consciousness and how our mind-stream acts as a carrier for both biographical and non-biographical traumas that are locked into the Healing Field of family, ancestral and past life memory. The same culture is also self-limited by its refusal to acknowledge the reality of the energy field in which these traumas, as well as those of our biographical timeline, are stored. And yet anyone can gain firsthand experience of the operation of these fields by simply engaging in one of the related therapies. Alternatively they can merely observe the operation of the Healing Field by attending, as a participant-observer, a few sessions of Family Constellations Therapy. As we will see in the next section, Constellation Therapy offers an ideal platform to observe at first hand the operation of the Healing Field.

The Family Nexus & the Ancestral Realm

Family Constellations is a unique form of therapy developed by Bert Hellinger from an amalgam of family therapy and traditional African healing practices[1]. Like family therapy it sees the family as the context for understanding personal issues. But unlike conventional therapy, it views this family context as possessing deep roots reaching back into the ancestral past and transmitting an influence down to the present day.

It's been many years now since my first experience with Family Constellations but I will never forget the impression that first session had on me. I felt as though the scales had dropped from my eyes. Attending the session with my wife we had no idea whatsoever about what to expect. We had gone along to discover what it was all about. We found ourselves in a large room with about

20 other people – most of whom we did not know and who, with few exceptions, did not appear to know each other.

The therapist asked who would like to work on a specific problem. One member of the group briefly stated their problem, giving very few details. The therapist then invited them to select people from the group to represent key aspects of their issue and position them in a way that intuitively represented the dynamics of the situation. This included selecting someone to represent themselves. After placing the representatives, the person was asked to sit on the sideline and observe what was about to take place.

Having been selected I was now standing within the group of people in the middle of the room. Something extraordinary now began to unfold. Whilst remaining fully conscious and self-aware I became subject to what I can only describe as an 'emotional overlay', a strong secondary emotion, mental attitude and physical posture that had nothing whatsoever to do with me – except, of course, the fact that I was experiencing them, but rather like an outside observer rather than a full participant. It was a curious state of being oneself and another person all at the same time! As the sessions progressed we began to realize that these secondary emotions, thoughts and physical reactions reflected those of the persons that we were, unknowingly, representing. Moreover, it made no difference whether that person was still alive, absent, missing or long dead. It was with these secondary characteristics that the constellation therapist worked to untangle, in some cases, age old conflicts involving family betrayals, abuse, deception and indeed all of the sordid twists and turns that constitute ancestral baggage. Another extraordinary thing was that as each conflict was resolved – in just the way that this would happen if the actual people were present by sincere apology and heartfelt forgiveness – the quality of the energy that we experienced changed. It became less jagged, less fraught with strong negative emotions until, at last, it resolved itself into an atmosphere of harmony and peace. This account describes the mechanics of the process but does not touch the 'inner life' of this profound process. For that we need to turn to a real case. The following account was provided by a close friend, Maureen, and details one of her constellations.

"In placing my family members, I had placed the people representing my father and sister together and separate from the people representing my mother and myself. The person who represented my mother stood, looking at the floor as if searching for something. The person who represented me was standing next to her, her hands held out as though waiting to receive something. The therapist asked the mother what she was looking for. She said there had to be more babies. The therapist told me that this meant that there were dead babies that needed to be acknowledged and she started throwing pillows on the floor to represent them. The mother was not satisfied and kept saying "There are more, there are more", but there were already many pillows on the floor. Then suddenly the therapist asked me if any of the babies had been born. My mother had had a baby while we lived in Nigeria and it had died one day later. The therapist brought someone else to stand before the mother and said 'Here is your daughter. Look at her. See her'. I think it was at this point in the session that things turned around for me because the mother said 'I can't look at her because I never saw her'. I was shocked. This woman who didn't even know my mother was talking with her mannerisms, saying things the way she would say them and now she was telling us she had never seen the baby. It was true. My mother had never seen her last daughter. Then the therapist began to line up women behind the mother. Grandmothers, their mothers, their mothers ... tracing the lineage of women in our family on my mother's side. About eight women down the line, she came across the 'blockage' in the female energy. As I watched I understood that the fear I had had since the birth of my son, the fear that he was certain to die, was not mine but energy carried through the women in the family and I was standing with my arms open to accept it. There and then I decided that I was not going to accept that energy. The therapist put me directly into my own role in the constellation and I refused to accept the fear. A couple of weeks following the session my fear for my son had almost disappeared."

To anyone attending a constellation it is quite clear that we are dealing with a field effect. The sensations of energy within the constellation are quite tangible. Once a constellation has been formed it is as though the feelings and emotional tone related to the people being represented exist timelessly and are re-constituted at that specific time and place by the re-enactment of a symbolic structure representing them. So accurate is this representation that if a key member of the field be left out – perhaps they were an unknown participant in this drama – then the field will indicate their absence and their place within the constellation. In other words the 'consciousness slice' of that time and place is interwoven timelessly within a field that continues to exert its influence down through its living descendants. For this reason it has been called the 'knowing field'[2].

Within the constellation we feel this energy in terms of both the overall emotional tone of the constellation and the specific feelings of the individual that we are representing. The energy is tangible. If we conduct a number of constellations during a single day we will soon begin to experience the classic symptoms of high energy – our head will feel 'full' or pressured. In this context it is, perhaps, worth mentioning that various types of intense energy work can lead to an uncomfortable concentration of energy in the head. Such a build-up manifests as sensations of fullness or pressure. On occasion it can lead to headaches. We may also experience similar difficulties if we have studied or concentrated on something for too long and feel too mentally restless to be able to relax. The reason for this is that due to the natural constriction presented by the neck any increase in the flow of inner energy circulates much less readily and tends to build-up in the head leading to a sensation of pressure. The standard solution to all such problems is a greatly simplified version of the classic Chinese Qi Gong meditation known as the 'Lesser Microcosmic Orbit'. The full meditative practice circulates the energy along the major meridians that run from the top of the head down the front of the body before turning under the base of the spine and ascending back to the top of the head via the spine. The shortened version of this meditation only utilizes the meridian that runs down the front of the body. The following steps will clear most sensations of mental restlessness and pressure:

- In a relaxed way, place your tongue on the roof of your mouth
- Visualize the activity/fullness/pain in your head as a heavy, slow moving liquid – like honey
- Visualize it moving down through your head across the bridge of the tongue, down the throat, chest & stomach & into the Hari Point which is just beneath the navel
- Place your hand on this point to retain mental contact with it
- Clear your mind of everything else

You will need to maintain this meditation for at least 10 minutes after which you will begin to feel relief from any discomfort. You will know that the meditation is complete because the release of energy from the head will leave you feeling mentally light and pleasantly empty. That this technique works so effectively is yet further proof that when we talk of inner energy, energy fields and morphic or knowing fields, we are describing real energy fields, not metaphorical ones.

One of the educational aspects of Family Constellations is the light that it throws on ageless values. Once each person's discordant feelings are reconciled, the quality of the emotion they have been experiencing changes for the better and the overall atmosphere becomes more harmonious. In the day to day life of the person for whom the constellation was performed old fears, illnesses and relationship issues fade away and are replaced by a renewed sense of energy and purpose. Time and again we see cases where healing only becomes possible when some past injustice is forgiven. The knowing field is not, therefore, just a passive carrier of neutral information. It is also an ethical field that cannot be 'fooled'; re-coding it requires real, and not feigned, repentance and forgiveness. When this happens the energy shifts, signaling the commencement of the healing process. The identification of ethics as a defining characteristic of these extended fields of consciousness is vitally important. The way that we behave now has profound ethical implications not only for ourselves and the people we affect. It has profound implications 'downstream', for our descendants and for their descendants. Given that these fields are ethical, the implications of our collective action, as families, communities, societies and, indeed, as a global culture, will resonate through time affecting the harmony and spiritual evolution of the entire planet. We will return to this crucial issue in the final chapter. We now need to draw out the implications of these cases for our understanding of healing, energy and consciousness.

Past lives

For many years Gulcan has been running voluntary workshops using energy psychology in major organizations. Amongst the thousands of cases the following one stands out,

"On a hot summer day, I was teaching Emotional Freedom Techniques (EFT) to a group of bank employees. One of the participants, who sat right in the front, challenged me by saying, "You know, I only joined the class because it was paid for by the bank. I don't think this is going to work. I am an engineer and this tapping thing looks ridiculous to me." I asked, "What is the problem, if you don't mind sharing it with the class?" He said that he had had an intense fear of heights since childhood. He added, "My wife is a psychiatrist. We have tried everything, but I can't even look down a flight of stairs." I asked, "OK, do you want to try to clear it with EFT now?" He nodded. I asked him to imagine himself somewhere high up. The moment he closed his eyes he started shouting, "My body is destroyed! My body is in pieces!" He was having difficulty breathing and we tapped for a few minutes until he calmed down. Then I felt like switching to use Tapas Acupressure Technique (TAT). When I made him repeat the phrase "All of the origins of this fear are healing now", he recovered the following memory. He was in his twenties. He was on top of a skyscraper, walking along the edge. He was not sure if he would jump off or not. He was not sure if he wanted to live. All of a sudden, a gust of wind caused him to lose his balance and fall. Holding the TAT pose he remembered he was looking down at his body, from about a meter above it. He was screaming that his body was in pieces. We finished the session by using TAT to affirm that that life and its experience of death was over; that he could enjoy his current life and that he was safe and secure. We also affirmed that heights were safe, unless he took unreasonable risks. The whole session took around twenty minutes and at the end of it he was able to go to the top of the building and look down four floors to the car park. He could not believe that he was now able to do this. For the first time in his life, he felt no fear at all. Walking down the stairs, he kept insisting that he was an engineer and that he did not believe in past lives. I said, "You know, I am an engineer, too. You do not have to believe in anything. It only matters that you can now look down the stairs so comfortably while we are talking". He asked me if his phobia would come back and I told him that it would not. He was so happy he left the class to go and celebrate with his wife."

Past lives or 'past lives'? Therapeutically it makes no difference. A trauma or phobia is real no matter what its cause, or seeming lack of one. Traces of past lives can emerge as key factors in any kind of energy work. Although there is an ongoing debate about the validity of recovered memories, there is little debate about the healing associated with their integration. An important point here is that unlike the various forms of past-life work or regression therapy, the cases that we come across are neither sought out nor induced. They emerge spontaneously as a natural part of a person's healing process. The following story relates another of Gulcan's cases.

"Alison, a woman in her early thirties came for help with a relationship problem. She was blonde and tall, with bright eyes though a bit of shy. She had double major, in civil engineering and physics. She described her problem as being "Stuck in a vicious circle of failed relationships". Apparently she was always looking for a physically specific type of partner, one that she described as "Having a broad chin and looking handsome". But every person she took up with turned out to be highly problematic so that all of these relationships were doomed from the start. I suspected that she was specifically attracted to problematic people in order to avoid lasting relationships and any possibility of marriage. Although her last "broad chinned, handsome looking" date did not want to have a relationship with her, she insisted that it could be made to work somehow. "I'm hoping that he will change and want to marry me. His looks are exactly those of the person I want," she said. She also said that she experienced an intense fear of loneliness, of being without a partner or marriage. She started using the meridian therapy techniques as she worked through these insights and as she did so her fears began to emerge. The last fear to come up was "I am afraid of marriage" and "he's going to leave me alone". We then started to clear these. The problem was defined as "I am afraid to get married". As she applied the technique to herself she sensed that something very sad had happened and after that she did not want to get married. She could not recall any event but she felt very down. She started to treat herself using the protocol "All the origins of this problem are healing now". At this point in my mind's eye I saw the interior of a small mosque. It was green inside and full of people praying. But when I told her this she said that it didn't mean anything to her. When she started to treat herself using the protocol "All the origins of this problem are healing in all of my past lives" she started crying vehemently. She said that she could 'see' herself in a small village, wearing a local gown and stirring food in a kitchen. Now the strange thing about these 'memories' is that they bore no relationship whatsoever to her upbringing, her scientific education or her sophisticated life and career in a big city. As she continued with the protocol the village woman that she identified with, was having very bad feelings about her husband. She remembered his name, Mehmet, and could even 'see' him. He was handsome and had a broad chin. With this memory she found herself filled with joy and excitement. But all of a sudden her mood changed and she felt intense fear. She reported that in this village life they had only been married for a couple of months before he had had to go away to war. Next she 'saw' a big crowd of people coming to the door of her village house to tell her that he had been killed along with two other men from the village. Then she saw the same small mosque that I had seen earlier but with three coffins inside it. At this point she experienced immense sorrow and pain in her neck and back, and then throughout her whole body. We worked through these feelings using another meridian therapy technique to clear them. Whilst doing this she said "loneliness is my destiny" and "I can't go on, I'm in too much pain. I want to leave my body, I can't endure this pain!" We then cleared these pains and emotions as well. After she had calmed down she said that even though she did not believe in past lives, she was sure that this was real. It was a past life trauma carried forward into the day to day drama of her relationships in this life. Next I used kinesiology to ask some questions about what had happened in and around the funeral. It seemed as though she had died traumatically at her husband's funeral and the trauma of these events had become 'locked in' to her energy body. After clearing all of her negative thoughts and feelings we started to work with positive affirmations such as "that life is over now" and "my new destiny is to have a happy relationship and marriage". I made her imagine what it would be like to be in a happy relationship and marriage. The client was delighted with the session. She said that it was the first time ever she could imagine herself married. The broad chinned Mehmet she had been looking for all this time now seemed to be just a distant and blurred memory. She no longer felt anything about him. She said that she had experienced a great liberation in her life. Her horizons opened and in her relationships she found that she was able to relate to men in new and more positive ways. In fact, she was introduced to four men within a week and chose one of them."

All of the past life cases that we have seen have arisen in the context of healing some ongoing problem that appeared to have no basis in the person's biographical time-line. The search for past lives is not something that is aimed at. It is just something that comes up in a certain percentage of cases as a by-product of resolving some acute and persistent personal issue. In such cases the problems experienced in this life are directly associated with traumatic events that appear to have occurred just before experiencing death in a past life. It is as though the trauma of these unresolved issues becomes 'locked into' a person's 'mind stream' and carried forward from life to life. In most of these cases it is impossible to prove conclusively that a past life was involved. Nevertheless most of these cases strike you with their vividness and a strong sense of real events lying behind them, events that continue to influence people's lives and behavior today.

A rebirthing breathwork client of mine had had an intense interest in ballet from early in life. When first taken to see a ballet she had burst into tears, overwhelmed by the familiarity and intensity of the experience. All through her life she had believed in reincarnation and that in one life she had been a ballerina. We commenced the session and the client, a regular meditator, was able to access a very high level of internal energy that produced sensations of ecstatic bliss. But all of a sudden the atmosphere changed. It was as though the session was thrown, suddenly and unexpectedly, into an intense tragedy. Her entire being - emotional and physically appeared to be consumed by the 'experience' of having 'lost her legs'. After integrating these difficult emotions, the client had a sense of a separate lifetime, of being a ballerina who had just discovered that she had lost her legs in an accident, though how this happened was not apparent. At the end of the session the client felt uplifted and revitalized. She said that she had always believed in reincarnation but that now she knew it to be a fact and understood it in a far more profound way. Later research revealed that a famous ballerina, Adele Granzow, had lost her legs in an accident in Berlin. But for the accident she would have been the first Swanilda, the main character in the ballet Coppelia, which places these events around 1869. I am not aware of any other ballerina that these tragic events could refer to.

The benefit that people seek and take away from such sessions is never the satisfaction of idle curiosity. It is the integration of some obscure but problematic aspect of their day to day lives. This integration leads to a deep and positive shift in their mental, emotional and physical lives. Recurrent situations, such as conflicts with authority figures or patterns of negative relationships, suddenly end and they experience a profound transformation and improvement in their quality of life.

Notes

1. *Hellinger, B. (1998) Love's Hidden Symmetry: What Makes Love Work in Relationships*
2. *Term coined by Dr. Albrecht Mahr*

Chapter 5

The Healing Field

Our Findings

We will first summarize our findings concerning the healing processes that we have covered up to now. Although they constitute only a tiny subset of the thousands of cases that we have dealt with on a daily basis for the last 15 years or so, they are typical. We will then go on to look for independent scientific confirmation of these ideas. The experiential evidence is clear and unambiguous. A range of biofield energies exist that lay outside those acknowledged by mainstream science. These fields are deeply implicated in all mental, physical and emotional health issues and in all effective healing processes.

Disciplines and practices for using these energies underlay the world's many natural healing, martial and spiritual traditions. They have done so for millennia. Despite this, even the possibility of the existence of such energies is largely ignored by mainstream science. This is due in large part to the common prejudice that these traditions are the products of a scientifically unsophisticated, pre-modern phase of humanity's evolution. On this reading the survival of these ideas into the modern age is only due to the slower pace of development in those countries were such traditions have persisted. Needless to say this common prejudice is only sustainable by ignoring the available research.

Biofield energies form cocoon-like fields around all life forms. Somewhat like the phenomenon of blind sight – the ability of the physically blind to sense the properties of objects – these fields are not perceptible to mechanical perception but are perceptible to the psychically gifted or as a result of inner cultivation. Disharmony within these fields arises as a result of mental, physical and emotional trauma and stress. Since these energy fields represent a more fundamental level of existence, healing on this level is disproportionately more effective.

Natural healers receive information that is critical to the healing process through empathic engagement. This deeper level of engagement is not just a passive, receptive state of mind. And the insights it gives rise to are not guesswork. It is a dynamic, empathic opening of one's humanity to understanding and helping another person. The healer's empathy is also an energetic state. Reaching out to and interacting with another person is to shift awareness and energetically interact with their energy field. It is through the medium of this shift that the healer may become aware of information that proves critical to the healing process. This intuitively derived information has a number of specific attributes:

a) It is often represented symbolically or pictorially, it may involve 'hearing' a name or seeing an object that is intimately related to a specific traumatic event
b) It may initially appear to be irrelevant, both to the healer and to the client
c) It provides the key that enables a client re-connect to a past trauma
d) It emerges at just the right time to facilitate the healing process

The important point here is that this information must be stored or held somewhere. Although it is private information, so private, in fact, that the client may have completely forgotten it or be otherwise unconscious of it, it is nevertheless accessible in the context of healing. Because of this, we have little alternative but to suppose that this information resides in an information bearing field connected with the client. The healer's intention to help is sufficient to facilitate a shift of awareness that allows the unconscious retrieval of information from the client's field. The act of 'playing back' that information to the client allows them to remember and re-connect with their feelings about any event underlying their problem. Once this past (distressed) energy state has been 'activated', energy psychology techniques can then be used to clear the distress. As we noted previously, the efficacy of these energy psychology techniques, even with the most intractable of problems, can be as high as 90%.

The healer's intention and desire to facilitate healing provides sufficient 'navigation', for want of a better word, of the client's consciousness field for the retrieval of relevant information. This is clearly a reversed or goal governed process. It starts from the goal – the intent of healing – and works to directly retrieve the information that will initiate or facilitate it. This type of goal governed, reverse causation is called 'teleological'. As the scientific method was developed during the 15th - 16th centuries, teleological forms of causation were rejected as contrary to the newly emerging scientific understanding. Mainstream science is founded on a view of causality based on reductionist materialism. All phenomena can be explained in terms of their emergence from interactions between smaller units of matter. From this perspective the existence of abstract 'end states' or 'goals' that dictate behaviors and outcomes at lower levels is simply 'unscientific'. Although this point of view has been challenged recently by such major figures in the philosophy of science as Thomas Nagel[1], it nevertheless remains the orthodoxy within mainstream science.

Robust evidence from remote viewing, dowsing and energy healing points quite clearly to the existence of teleological processes that, given some goal or objective, work backwards to retrieve relevant information. In the context of healing this process depends heavily upon the personal qualities of healers and their ability to connect empathically with their clients. Such capabilities are not, therefore, evenly distributed amongst the population nor are they readily repeatable. For this reason they tend to elude formal investigation. Nevertheless, once developed and honed, this faculty works reliably to facilitate healing and integration. Extensive practical experience indicates this 'teleological faculty' stands alongside, and fully equal to, our analytic faculty for discerning material causation. Given the thrust of modernity over the centuries, and specifically its neglect of inner cultivation in favor of instrumentalism, our faculty for direct knowing has been neglected and under-developed.

It is important to stress that these processes do not involve guesswork. Guesswork requires effort. It tends to proceed by placing the available information in some context and trying to work out what the missing parts could be. But with the spontaneous emergence of information that facilitates the healing process the right information emerges spontaneously at the right time. We now need to move on to examine the information and affect bearing fields within which the healing process takes place.

The Deep Structures of Consciousness

The accounts of healing that we have covered during the last two chapters entail the existence of a number of layers or strata of integrated information and emotional affect. In most conventional accounts three to four layers of consciousness are recognized: present moment awareness, biographical memory and the biographical unconscious (forgotten and suppressed biographical material). These layers constitute the Personal Field of Consciousness. Optionally, a collective layer is sometimes recognized. This is the 'collective unconscious' defined by Carl Jung. It acts as a repository for the shared 'archetypal' material that recurs throughout human cultural history and structures processes of profound personal transformation. But to account for the experiences associated with the cases that we have been exploring we need to add at least four, and possibly more, 'fields of consciousness'. The existence of these extra layers is a challenge to, if not a refutation of, the mainstream understanding that consciousness only arises during the final three months prior to birth[2]. Two of these extra layers enhance our model of the Personal Field of Consciousness. The other two are collective layers of consciousness. Together I call these fields The Healing Field (or The Healing Fields) since they are regularly implicated in cases of healing, especially once the healer is aware of or attuned to their existence. Many cases of failure to effect healing are attributable to a failure to connect with disturbances held within these fields. The first two (personal) fields within The Healing Field are:

The Field of Perinatal Memory. Forgotten and suppressed fetal memories during which our experience is, in certain respects, inseparable from that of our mother. It is 'biographical', its affects constitute a vital part of our identity, but at the same time it is shared with and indistinguishable from our mother's experience. This area has been extensively researched by the psychiatrist and one of the founders of the Transpersonal movement in psychology, Stanislav Grof[3]. The emergence of perinatal memories is usually associated with a variety of energy healing techniques such as rebirthing breathwork or any of the meridian therapy techniques.

The Field of Past Life Memory. An extended biographical time line encompassing past lives. This layer manifests as bodily defects, health and relationship issues that can be traced directly to traumatic deaths in previous lives. These cases have been extensively researched by the psychiatrist, Ian Stevenson[4,5]. The emergence of past life memories is usually associated with Past Life Regression Therapy but also tend to surface in the context of a variety of energy healing modalities such as rebirthing breathwork or those involving any of the meridian therapy techniques.

The other two fields (collective) fields within the Healing Field are:

The Field of the Family Unconscious. An inherited field that affects the members of the immediate family. We have seen that siblings often 'inherit' an unconscious guilt concerning a dead sibling or are burdened with the effort to 'live' a dead sibling's life in addition to their own – even when the sibling died before they were born and they were consciously unaware of their ever having existed. These types of issue typically manifest in the context of Family Constellation Therapy associated with its originator, psychiatrist Bert Hellinger[6]. They also surface in other forms of energy healing, especially those involving the use of meridian therapy techniques.

The Field of the Ancestral Unconscious. Another inherited field that affects the members of the extended, multi-generational family. It manifests as emotional, physical and relationship issues that can be directly traced to unresolved traumas and injustices in the ancestral line. These types of affect are typically surfaced in the context of Family Constellation Therapy.

It is important to note that the idea of these additional fields did not emerge from theoretical or philosophical considerations.

They emerged in an attempt to explain recurrent cases of healing that hinged on information and traumatic affects from beyond a person's biographical timeline. When these affects were integrated they triggered the healing of present day emotional and physical problems that had otherwise persisted through many attempts to deal with them. The existence of these fields, and especially the collective fields, goes far towards confirming the overall 'field-like' nature of consciousness and the reality of the 'extended mind'. But unlike the philosopher's 'extended mind'[7], which is only 'extended' in as much as physical media (diaries and electronic media) can capture information, this 'extended mind' is the real article – it is extended in a quite literal sense. Just how far-reaching are these fields – how far does consciousness, and therefore the potential reach of our awareness, extend?

If Family Constellations Therapy allows us to trace a continuum of consciousness back in time to encompass the experiences of distant ancestors, how far do these fields of consciousness extend? The Global Consciousness Project[8] is a large scale experiment to attempt to answer this question. The experiment involves a worldwide network of random number generators connected to computers. These create a stream of random data in which no underlying structure can be discerned. A program extracts this data and forwards it to a central database for analysis. The idea is that if a global consciousness field exists, during any major event that engages people's attention globally, this should show up as a disturbance in the random flow of data. Randomness should give way to the sudden emergence of order and coherence in the data. It has been found that major events, such as the attacks on the World Trade Center in 2001, appear to be accompanied by distinctive surges in ordered activity in the 1 to 2 hours before and after they occur. Whilst the conclusions drawn from this ongoing experiment remain controversial, it is a distinctive possibility that the whole planet is embedded in a responsive field that is sensitive to meaningful activity. Can the planet's resonance and our own mental activity be connected? An experienced meditator offered me this account of her experimentation along these lines,

"It occurred to me one day that the Earth itself might be a frequency that I could meditate with. I started to meditate with this in mind and found that I started to experience a state of what can only be described as global or planetary consciousness. This peaceful, harmonious state was quite distinct from the normal meditative states that I was used to."

We can summarize our findings concerning the strata or layers that we have encountered within The Healing Field with a simple diagram depicting the 4 Personal Fields of Consciousness closest to our day to day awareness and the 2 Collective Fields of Consciousness associated with us (diagram below). Please note, I am making no claims about the completeness of this model. I am merely stating that these fields are apparent in healing contexts where they act as the repositories of traumas that affect our mental, physical and emotional health and well-being. The final point that we need to reaffirm is that these fields can be interrogated by complete strangers, as in Family Constellation Therapy. They are not, therefore, 'in our heads'.

Diagram III: The fields of consciousness

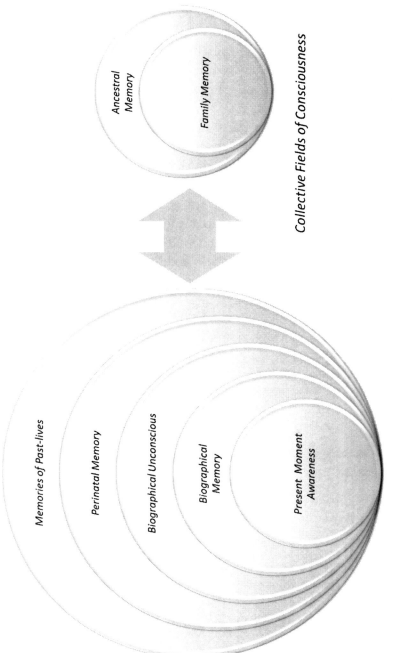

The Morphic Field

The second step that we wanted to accomplish was to see if we could find independent confirmation for these ideas. The founder of Family Constellation therapy, Burt Hellinger, has written,

"The first phenomenon ... is that there is obviously a dimension of awareness that we all share. We all participate in a common field. The representatives often feel and behave like the actual persons they represent"[9].

To better understand this 'shared dimension of awareness' Hellinger refers to the work of biologist Dr. Rupert Sheldrake[10]. We have already reviewed some of Sheldrake's research (Chapter 2). We now need to examine the conclusions that can be drawn from this research and how they relate to our own findings.

In biology, morphogenesis is the name for the process governing the spatial development and organization of living organisms. The word comes from the combination of the Greek words *morphe* (form) and *genesis* (coming into being). Historically there has been a back and forth debate concerning the respective merits of genetic versus 'field' explanations of how morphogenesis works. Swimming against the tide of today's mainstream scientific opinion Rupert Sheldrake has argued that purely genetic explanations fail to explain key aspects of organized growth that can be demonstrated to be the results of field effects.. One of the major problems for his approach is that the nature of the relevant fields is not readily apparent. Whilst it is common knowledge that all living organisms emit a whole range of electromagnetic fields, it is by no means clear whether Sheldrake's morphogenetic fields are electromagnetic in nature or not. In chapter three we introduced the concept of 'vital' or 'subtle' energies and mainstream science's rejection of them. Sheldrake's morphogenetic fields may also be of this nature. He describes them as, "physical in the sense that they are a part of nature, though they are not yet mentioned in physics books"[11].

Sheldrake has further extended the concept of morphogenetic

fields beyond their immediate biological context to explain the emergence of organized behavior at all levels of life and culture. To distinguish this expanded conception from the narrower biological one Sheldrake calls these fields 'Morphic fields', and explains their function as one of organizing,

> "the form, structure and patterned interactions of systems under their influence – including those of animals, plants, cells, proteins, crystals, brains and minds."[12]

Sheldrake attributes three fundamental purposes to Morphic Fields. Firstly, they carry information that provides the environmental input that conditions the development of all living systems. Secondly, they act as a medium of information exchange that coordinates life forms and facilitates learning even when species are physically isolated from one another. Thirdly, they condition behavior and cultural trends and provide a plausible mechanism for such ideas as units of cultural transmission (memes[13]) or the transmission of values (vMemes[14]).

All of these 'top-down' processes are said to occur through a form of causality he calls 'Morphic Resonance'. We have all experienced a sense of wonder at the coordination of vast flocks of birds or shoals of fish moving with perfect synchronization at high speed as though they were of 'one mind'. These displays have the characteristics of being embedded in, and responsive to, a field that unifies and harmonizes their activities. Experiments indicate that whenever a life-form develops a particular quality or ability, all of the other members of that life-form, no matter where they are in the world, become capable of developing the same quality or capability in much less time than the first members, despite the fact that they have shared no physical interaction[15]. This 'communication at a distance' can only be due to the existence of a shared information-bearing field.

These ideas share distinctive parallels, if not identities, with those emerging from the field of energy healing. Information relating to past lives, family and ancestral history (before one's birth) can only be derived from The Healing Field, the transpersonal field in which it resides. Experience shows that in addition The Healing Field also holds the emotional affects that accompanied the original events. These affects exist as disharmonies within the fields. As such they continue to reverberate down to the present day affecting the health and well-being of new members of the same group. Given that this disharmony arises from personal and social injustice, harmony can only be re-established when re-dress has been obtained. We will return to this theme, the ethical nature of the fields, and the implication of this in the final chapter.

Beyond The Healing Field

Recently two philosophers reflecting on the implications of Sheldrake's theories speculated,

> "If he had confined himself to examining the mores of migrating butterflies or of homing pigeons, he might have encountered less criticism … just how commonsensical is it to believe, for example, that rituals have an existence in some sort of physical sense - a field that is built up by continued activity. Is there, somewhere, a morphic field of Masonic rites?"[16]

Do organizations possessing historical continuity and consistent patterns of ritual practice generate a collective field of memory, ritual and symbol? Amongst magical orders the generation of such fields has always been recognized as one of the main purposes of ritual activity. Such 'artificial' collective fields of shared symbols and energies are called 'egregores'. By undertaking certain shifts in awareness (for example, out of body experiences or OBEs) it is possible to 'visit' these collective 'dreamscapes'. This is especially the case when meditative practice is combined with changes in the level and intensity of our life-energy. It was such a shift that gave rise to the experiences recounted below.

"Our Reiki teacher, Hale, possessed a strong inner energy. Anomalous phenomena often manifested around her. She put this down to the fact that she frequently experienced the rising of kundalini energy. Kundalini is the name given to the store of life-energy at the base of the spine. Increasing the level of activation of this energy is the objective of most systems of spiritual yoga. Completely activated it gives rise to experiences of enlightened awareness. In the course of rising, kundalini triggers a range of 'siddhis' or psychic powers. I suspect that it was the intensity of Hale's energy that led to the strange visionary experiences recounted below. These experiences occurred during a group meditation involving 7 to 8 people that we undertook with her.

"During the meditation, like a vivid dream, I became aware that I was standing in a hall. The floor consisted of black and white squares arranged like a chessboard. On the floor to my right lay a coffin and, curiously enough, I saw that I was laying in it. A railway track led past it to the left and entered a dark tunnel. I followed this track and entered the tunnel. As I moved through it, the tunnel bent upwards and I found myself entering a pool of bright light that was so intense that I couldn't make out any detail. It is difficult to express depth of feeling, of a sense of homecoming and acceptance that I experienced there. Afterwards, when I shared my experience, I found that she too had had a near identical experience – the same checkered floor, coffin, railway line and tunnel. How we could 'share' the same bizarre surroundings in a meditative state?

In a subsequent meditative state she made out some additional features of this strange environment. It contained a lectern from which a long tongue descended like a red carpet being unrolled and a booming voice saying "A well hung tongue". This strange expression puzzled both of us. Neither of us had any idea what it meant or referred to. Nor is it one that would naturally occur to most native speakers, let alone someone for whom English is their second or third language. You can imagine my amazement when, some months later, reading a nonfiction book by the novelist Andrew Sinclair exploring the lives of his knightly ancestors, I came across the following obscure lines from the initiation rite of an 18[17] century Scottish Masonic lodge,

Question: Which is the Kye of your Lodge? (trans: what is the key of your lodge?)

Answer: A well hung tongue

Now whilst this usage can be fairly described as strange, it is even stranger that it should spontaneously occur to someone of a different country and culture with no knowledge of, interest in or involvement with masonry. Those who study such things will have recognized the checkered floor as characteristic of Masonic Lodge rooms worldwide and the coffin as a recognized symbol of the third degree or Master Mason, a degree that enacts the symbolic death and resurrection of the candidate."

What is it that happens during meditation? And how can the semi-secret imagery and practices of Freemasonry spontaneously occur to people who have no relationship with the order, and certainly not in an 18th century Scottish guise? Given that all of this emerged spontaneously, that it occurred, independently, to two people with no connection with masonry, across a geographical and cultural divide and that it involved accurate references to obscure symbolism and ritual phrases, how can we explain it? The archetype of the Masonic lodge room and its rituals, as well as that of other secret societies, exist on a subtler level of reality, one that is accessible via certain altered states. But if these systems exist as morphic fields, what of their resonance effects?

"This experience was not, however, just a shared visual theatre. It was to have a deep and unexpected dynamic. It was connected with a profound shift that I experienced shortly after in the nature and quality of my self-perception and understanding. A shift that I can only explain as a relativization of my ego based selfhood in favor of a broader 'witnessing' selfhood. The most obvious external marker of this shift was that I freely and easily abandoned my many years long enjoyment of tobacco and alcohol. I just felt that I no longer needed them, that they were not healthy and that I should simply abandon them. If I still wanted these things, the larger "I" that I now had access to simply forbade them, they were not "good" for the smaller, desiring "I". This 'relativization of the ego' has remained to this day. And this, surely, is the point of the initiation. It enacted this process symbolically by representing the candidate as having died only to be 'resurrected', brought back to life and lifted up to proceed on a 'higher', that's to say, more aware and less instinctively reactive trajectory in life."

We need to pursue these issues further by examining even more extreme and anomalous experiences. We will seek to answer the question, what else does the 'public space' of the collective fields of consciousness contain? For example, what other forms of awareness may operate within it? Once again, advanced healing practices turn up some unusual presences.

Notes

1. Nagel, T. (2012) *Mind and Cosmos : Why the Materialist Neo-Darwinian Conception of Nature is Almost Certainly False* p.6667, 9193

2. Koch, C. *'When Does Consciousness Arise?' Scientific American,* September / October 2009

3. Grof, S. (1992) *The Holotropic Mind: The Three Levels of Human Consciousness & How They Shape Our Lives*

4. Stevenson, I. *'Birthmarks and Birth Defects Corresponding to Wounds on Deceased Persons' Journal of Scientific Exploration,* Vol. 7, No. 4, pp. 403-410, 1993

5. Pasricha, SK., Keil, J., Tucker, JB. & Stevenson, I. *'Some Bodily Malformations Attributed to Previous Lives' Journal of Scientific Exploration,* Vol. 19, No. 3, pp. 359-383, 2005

6. Hellinger, B. (1998) *Love's Hidden Symmetry: what makes love work in relationships*

7. Clark, A. & Chalmers, DJ. *'The Extended Mind' Analysis* 58:10-23, 1998

8. http://noosphere.princeton.edu

9. Hellinger, B. *'The Phenomenological Approach in Psychotherapy'*

10. Sheldrake, R. (2009) *Morphic Resonance: The Nature of Formative Causation*

11. Sheldrake, R. *'Morphic Resonance & Morphic Fields: Collective Memory & the Habits of Nature' New Dawn Magazine,* Special Issue 15

12. ibid

13. Dawkins, R. (1976) *The Selfish Gene*

14. Beck, D. & Cowan, C. (1996) *Spiral Dynamics: Mastering Values, Leadership, and Change*

15. *Sheldrake, R. (1988) The Presence of the Past: Morphic Resonance and the Habits of Nature Ch.9*

16. *Rich, P. & Merchant, D. 'Rupert Sheldrake and the Search For Morphic Resonances' Contemporary Philosophy 22, 453-44 (2000)*

17. *Sinclair, A. (1993) The Sword and the Grail p. 165*

Chapter 6

Healing on extended planes

Extended Planes of Existence

"one man's ancestor is another man's ghost"[1]

Of all the chapters of this book, this one is the most challenging. I want to emphasize that I grew up in a staunchly secular, rationalist and humanist tradition. My academic training in the analytical tradition of Philosophy included formal logic, the theory of knowledge and the philosophy of science. It was rigorous, focused and entirely, for want of a better word, 'grounded'. The conclusions that I have come to in the intervening years and reported here have, so to speak, been 'forced upon me' by the sheer weight of practical experience arising from 35 years of experience with a range of energy based modalities and some 15 years of professional energy healing work. These conclusions go against everything that I had, until fairly recently, believed to be true of reality. I report these cases as they occurred. Some of them are disturbing. All of them pose a significant challenge to our commonsense conception of the borders of selfhood, autonomy and the underlying nature of reality.

Most of us think that what we see is all there is. Yet there is ample evidence that what we see is only a small fraction of what there is. That there is a gap between these two becomes apparent when we encounter individuals and entire cultures with fundamentally different perceptions of reality. The respected anthropologist, Edith Turner, has written about the conflict she experienced between her scientific training and her actual experience undertaking field work in a traditional society. One day, whilst attending a healing ritual she saw, emerging from the back of the woman who was being healed,

> "... a giant thing emerging out of the flesh of her back. This thing was a large, gray blob about six inches across, a deep gray opaque thing emerging as a sphere"[2].

She described it as,

> "a miserable object, purely bad, without any energy at all,

and much more akin to a restless ghost ... There is spirit stuff. There is spirit affliction; it is not a matter of metaphor and symbol, or even psychology." [3]

We will never know what, in this situation, facilitated the shift of awareness that allowed Edith Turner to 'see', at least for a short time, what was taking place on the deeper levels of the healing ritual. But this type of experience is neither rare and nor is it confined to the remotest regions of the world. It forms a regular part of the day to day experience of many energy-based healers worldwide. The segregation of these deeper layers of reality from our day to day perception leaves us with a skewed understanding of 'what there is' and what forces may be acting upon us.

We have already seen that most of us remain completely unaware and unsuspecting of the effects of unseen influences – family, ancestral, past life – on our health and well-being. These influences may be far more pervasive than most of us suspect. What follows is another of Gulcan's cases.

"I was staying with a friend and student whilst delivering a training course in her town. We prepared the couch for me to sleep on. But when I lay down I was overcome with an overwhelming sense of heaviness. I felt that someone had died there and that she had been unaware of the fact that she was dying. I felt an energy come over me. My student confirmed that everyone who visited her was overcome with similar feelings of heaviness and never stayed very long. I started talking to it saying, "You should go to the light. You will find healing there. Now go to the light". We then sent energy to the situation and prayed that whoever it was realize that they had died, that they were trapped between the worlds and that they could be healed by making their transition. After a little while the feelings of heaviness released and the atmosphere throughout the house brightened up. I learned later that the opposite neighbor's six year old son would never come in the house. He complained that an old lady across the street was continuously staring at him from the window of that room. Returning from the training the next day the driver recognized the address that we had given him and started to tell us about the old woman who used to live there. He told us that she had been bedridden laying in that room for many years before dying there."

Classically, hauntings are associated with the lingering attachment of 'deceased persons' to certain aspects of their incarnated lives. These include places or objects to which they were especially attached during life or with the manner and circumstances of their death. The idea of 'haunting', and the very category of 'deceased person', is troublesome in more ways than one. Modernity has no place for it or, indeed, anything else that upsets its positivist interpretation of reality. And yet, year in, year out, across the world these phenomena continue to be widely encountered and, in some cases, recorded. Although the phenomena of haunting is extremely elusive, it is nevertheless accessible to the psychically gifted and to those able to extend their awareness to encompass these extended planes of existence. The following experience, provided by Amanda, a close friend who is also a manager in major transnational corporation, illustrates just how extensive the phenomena can be in the wake of a major disaster. It is also significant in highlighting the healing work undertaken by certain esoteric groups.

"I had noticed a certain executive at work – we had a 'nodding' acquaintance – though what drew my attention to her I'm really not sure. We finally met thru a common friend and realized we had much in common with shared interests in spirituality, meditation and healing. Shortly after the big earthquake in Haiti, she approached me and asked if I wanted to help the people affected by it. I answered that of course I would. She then explained that she was a part of a larger group and that the nature of the help they provided was to assist people who had died unexpectedly and were still lingering, lost, on the Earth plane to make their transition. The help that was envisaged involved projecting myself onto the astral plane, gathering together those lost between the planes and bringing them to a certain place where their transition could take place.

That night, during my regular meditation, I intended to project to that dimension to help those in need. I found myself in a zone which was not of this Earth. There was a lack of light – it was an unearthly greenish-gray color – but I could still see. First I saw an old man. He was crying and looked scared and confused. His eyes were red from crying. He didn't know where he was or what had happened to him. He was sitting on the rubble next to a fire. Crying, he asked me where everyone else was. I told him that he was safe. I asked him to wait there for me to come back and that I would bring help. At this stage I had no clue what else to say. As I continued looking for others, I saw another old man, holding the hand of a 5-6 year old boy. It was his grandson. I knew they were both dead but the old man was still trying to rescue his grandson. My heart sank for them. I told him that he should wait until I came back. Next I saw an old lady. She was still under the rubble (in fact this was how she perceived her situation). I helped her remove the rubble. I felt that her lungs had collapsed. I helped her to sit up, brushed the dust from her clothes and did Reiki to her lungs until she felt better. I asked her to wait for me until I came back.

The next morning, the first thing I did was to share my experiences with my friend. At this point I wasn't even sure if I was making this up. I certainly didn't know how to help those people. She reassured me that my experience was valid and asked me to go back. She told me to do everything to convince them (if necessary to put a Red Cross vest on) to come with me. She then asked me to take them along a path to a park across from a large Library building. She told me that this is where the akashic records are kept. Once there, she asked me to invite the relatives and loved ones of those people to come and assist them to transition to the other side. I felt extremely nervous about attempting all of this. I didn't know if it would work or if I could really help them, but I had no choice but to try.

That night I returned to the same plane. It wasn't hard to find them. I told them I had good news and that I would take them to where they would be reunited with their families. It wasn't hard to convince them. I visualized the path and found myself across from the Library building. Their loved ones came one by one and led them away to the Library. The next day when I awoke I felt exhausted, I was completely drained and felt very sad. I still wasn't sure if all of this had been a real experience or not. I again shared my experience with my friend and she said that she had seen me outside the library but that I wasn't ready to see her and the other helpers who had gathered there. She explained that they use different methods to convince people to make their transition, including creating an elevator of light or a bridge. She confirmed that I would feel exhausted since I was operating on a plane for which I was not energetically prepared and had fully exposed myself to their emotions. It took me a couple days to regain my energy, but it had been really worth it."

Hauntings are not simple, unitary phenomena. There is no one explanation that covers all cases. Nor can they be understood solely in terms of their external manifestations - temperature fluctuations, electromagnetic anomalies and so on. Hauntings are also profoundly intensional patterns of activity. By 'intension', as distinct from 'intention', I refer to the cluster of concepts around our ideas of agency: deciding, intending, acting and so on - all of which give rise to meaning and, with that, ethical significance. This is a quite different order of understanding that cannot be reduced to some corresponding physical description. Classifying hauntings solely in terms of their external manifestation leaves this essential dimension, their real significance, untouched. It is the business of the healer to be aware of the intentional and ethical dimensions of all phenomena in order to be able to formulate an appropriate response. We can better understand this phenomena by distinguishing between different manifestations or 'types' of haunting:

a) Residual Hauntings. Residual hauntings manifest as an extremely narrow band of repeated behavior, movement or activity. They demonstrate remarkable consistency with people reporting similar experiences over long periods of time. They do not respond to or interact with the people who observe them. They behave, rather, like a short video clip that constantly replays. Because of this they are widely understood as a psycho-energetic imprint on the surroundings made whilst the person was still alive or the related events, such as a battle, were taking place.

b) Disoriented Hauntings. Disoriented hauntings are caused by deceased persons who are either unaware or uncomprehending of the fact that they have died. This can be due to their having experienced a sudden or unexpected death. They may exhibit a strong attachment to the places that they were familiar with when alive. They may also experience a strong sense that the living are intrusive on their privacy. The account that I gave at the start of this chapter concerning the old lady and the longer account concerning the earthquake both have elements that fit this category.

c) Petitionary Hauntings. Petitionary hauntings can arise as a result of a deceased person bearing an unfulfilled sense of personal responsibility for resolving some issue. The haunting may involve attempting to contact close friends or relatives who can resolve their unfinished business. Another of Gulcan's cases is relevant in this context.

"I was working on a client's personal issues using energy psychology when all of a sudden I felt something like energy come through me. I experienced a profound sense of sadness that made me feel like crying. Internally I heard the word 'inheritance'. I asked the client whether there was a problem with an inheritance and she immediately replied that there was. I had a sense of a person and asked her if this problem was related to a man. Again she replied that it was. I next sensed that there was an unfinished business relating to this inheritance and that the man was saying to my client "please, you must take over". My client said that she had immediately understood the significance of this exchange. She explained that her uncle had been a prominent lawyer who had helped bring her up. He was like a second father to her and they trusted each other implicitly. Since he was a respected figure, the family had entrusted their title deeds to him in order to ensure a fair distribution of the lands. Unfortunately he had died suddenly and unexpectedly before he could fulfil this responsibility. When the family asked for the title deeds his widow could find no trace of them. With that the matter had remained unresolved for years. Despite the urging of the deceased uncle, my client's first response was that she was afraid to take on such a difficult task."

Petitionary hauntings can also arise due to a deceased person's sense of injustice. Examples include, having their innocence recognized for a crime that they were accused of but which they did not commit or having someone who stole from them or was responsible for their death recognized as having done so. These hauntings often subside once the issues that concerned the deceased are addressed to their satisfaction.

d) Intercessory Hauntings. Intercessory hauntings arise as a result of a deceased person bearing a sense of personal responsibility for protecting or helping some person, usually a close relative. These hauntings also subside once the issues that concern the deceased have been addressed. In chapter 2 I gave an example of this type of haunting with Gulcan's case of helping a widow come to terms with her husband's death. In that case Gulcan had once again felt an energy coming through herself, picked up the image of a man doing the washing-up at a kitchen sink, strong feelings of sadness and the message "I don't want you to do this". This had helped the client to let go of trying to recover the comfort associated with her long, happy married life, to re-connect with her feelings concerning her loss and resolve the long standing sadness that had enveloped her.

Accounts like this challenge us on many different levels. Like the evidence from near death experiences and past lives, they strongly imply the continuity of, at least some degree of, conscious awareness, sense of responsibility and ethical judgment beyond death. From this point of view death is revealed to be a transitional state that involves the dissolution, over time, of the relative personality and its energetic supports in favor of a higher level identity sometimes called the mind-stream, Higher or Over Self. Traditional systems of spiritual cultivation provide detailed descriptions of this process[4]. Despite the vagueness surrounding the process of dying and sense of unreality associated with the postmortem or intermediate world, what is unquestioned is our ability to undertake healing on such extended planes.

In the context of oneonone healing the intercession of deceased persons sometimes forms an inseparable part of the healing process. We have already commented on the advanced retrocausal 'navigation' of the a-temporal, information-bearing field that the healer's intentionality brings about. To this we now need to add its openness to the voices and wishes of the deceased. In the context of healing this communication is always a positive contribution to the healing process. It may also allow for an unexpected reunion with the deceased that re-affirms their love and concern across the borders of death. Such interventions can be a major factor in facilitating the healing and closure, for the living as well as the dead, of years of pain, separation and loss.

Spirit/Entity Attachment

So far our accounts of interactions with deceased persons have focused on the purposeful phenomena that can arise spontaneously in the course of healing – even when that healing is taking place out of body. In these cases the healer is not deliberately setting out to act as a medium. Once the healing issue (and facilitating the transition of deceased persons is a form of healing) is resolved, any link or communication with the deceased ceases. But some attachments can be unwanted and intrusive presences in the lives of people with whom they have no connection, as the following case provided by a close friend illustrates,

"I am now 51 years old. Two major lifelong problems could have darkened my life forever. Because I chose transformation and healing, it has turned into a totally different journey. When I was a small child there was a period, starting from the age of 2 or

3 years old until I was 10, during which I was sexually abused by my uncle. Later, at 15 or 16 years of age I started drinking to tend the wounds inflicted by this abuse. This turned into a big alcohol problem. About 2000 I started to seek healing for both of these problems. I was able to get help through the use of energy psychology techniques combined with Alcoholics Anonymous. I made good progress but the alcoholism was difficult to manage and required a lot of self-discipline. During this journey I was introduced to Regression Therapy. I feel that my healing experience contains such valuable insights that I want to share them with you.

During a session with my regression therapist, after I had entered a trance, my therapist detected the presence of a spirit/entity attachment in my energy field. She was able to determine when it first attached itself to me. During my first experience of sexual abuse I had 'escaped' out of my body to get away from the pain of what was happening to me. The entity had attached itself to me at that time. Up until the regression session, for well over 40 years, I had had no idea that I had such an attachment. Nor would I have believed in the possibility of such a thing had I been told about it! My therapist was able to enter into a dialogue with the entity and an interesting story emerged. The spirit/entity had been an alcoholic and a prostitute who had lived in France. She had had a daughter. When her daughter was 3 years old, she herself had been murdered. Because of her sense of responsibility for her daughter she was unable to make her transition and had remained by her daughter's side throughout her life until her daughter died.

When I experienced my first sexual abuse and left my body, I was the same age as her daughter was when she had been murdered. As we noted earlier, it was during this experience that she attached herself to my energy field. The therapist later explained to me that every time these cases appeared there is always a positive intention behind the attachment. In this case the entity was trying to help me to cope with my emotional pain in the only way that she knew how, by using alcohol. After all, she had been an alcoholic herself. It then dawned on me that this helped to explain why I had been stealing alcohol from home and always looked for alcohol wherever I went.

The therapist convinced the entity to leave my energy field and to seek healing and find peace by making her transition.

When I opened my eyes I was amazed by what had happened. Because of the method used I remembered everything. Nothing had been imposed on me. That night I went to a dinner. I drank a little of the wine that was offered me but found that I couldn't even finish the glass! This was a first for me! Many addictions can be healed through regression therapy. Addiction can be a multi-layered problem, so people need to be patient. Not every case of addiction is associated with entity/spirit attachment. Six months have now passed since this healing. I have not had to make an effort not to drink alcohol. I would rate my need for alcohol at about zero."

If we wish to conceptualize this phenomenon a little more clearly it is helpful to distinguish between the different parts of the energy-body and understand how each is affected by the process of dying. The energy-body can be roughly divided between the lower frequency physical and etheric bodies and the higher frequency astral bodies and their emotional memories (leaving aside the complex issue of the basis for continuity from life to life and what happens to that). At death the physical/etheric and astral/emotional bodies separate. The physical body decomposes and over time its energetic support, the etheric body, dissolves. The astral bodies and their emotional charge and memories continue for some time before they too dissolve. On this model learned experience is transmuted upwards to form the basis for life-review and renewed incarnations. In rare cases this natural process can be subverted through the shock of unexpected or sudden death or because of obsessive attachment to aspects of incarnate experience. In such cases fragments of the astral body can remain connected to fragments of the etheric body and maintain a discrete existence[5].

> "Since the astral body contains desires and emotions, intense desires that were not transmuted or integrated during life may be released into the universal field, where they can wander or drift about as though looking for a vehicle through which to express themselves" [6].

'Express themselves' in this context means the parasitic attachment to and influence over the behavior of a living being. Such entities can sustain a virtual existence by feeding of the life-energy of the living. Most people subjected to this form of parasitism do not suspect that their health problems, feelings of lethargy, extreme emotions, dietary or sexual impulses are being manipulated by an external entity. For one thing modern culture distains the notion of such 'hidden' agency, that's to say, one that remains unseen by the average observer. For this reason the very awareness of this possibility and the skills necessary to discern and deal with it have largely atrophied in modern life. Based solely on their personal experience some clinical psychologists[7] and psychiatrists[8,9] have been forced to acknowledge the reality of spirit/entity attachment, understand its impact on mental and physical health and acquire the necessary skills to deal with it[10]. Nevertheless, in general modernity remains unwilling to acknowledge such lived realities. Such psycho-energetic fragments account for the majority (at least 99%) of the spirit/entity attachments known and recognized in every period and culture,

"It is probably such etheric-astral complexes that form the basis of discarnate entities known as Gui[11] in Chinese Medicine"[12] (diagram below).

The presence of spirit / entity attachment is often signaled by a persistent muscular stiffness, ache or pain or injuries that do not heal and for which there is no medical explanation. It may also be signaled by psychologically unaccountable addictions, compulsive dietary and sexual behaviors. It is important to emphasize that this phenomena is extremely rare. People who suffer from any of these symptoms need to work through regular medical and psychological processes, especially ones that incorporate the new energy psychology techniques, before they start to explore the possibility of spirit or entity attachment. If such attachments are found most experienced energy healers can easily remove them in one short session.

Diagram IV: An Etheric-Astral Complex or Gui

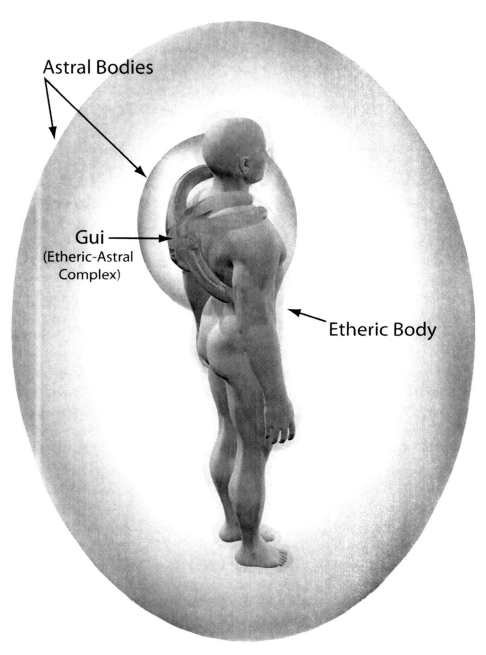

(Image courtesy of Michael & Richard Greenwood)

Spirit attachment occurs most often in situations where people are energetically vulnerable as a result of abuse, illness, injury or trauma. They can also arise as a result of exposure to extreme situations or places where anomalous phenomena are known to exist. Spirit attachment is especially associated with places where sudden death is common, such as hospitals. People who have recently undergone surgery or suffered an accident that required an operation under anesthesia may experience persistent problems that never seem to clear up. In such cases it is possible, though still very rare, that the remnant of a person who has recently died, has attached itself to their energy-body. When people become aware of these attachments they are experienced as intrusive, sometimes behaviorally manipulative and always parasitic upon their energy.

Other forms of entity attachment

"James, a fit, healthy young man who had recently completed his military service was referred to me for help. He had, quite literally, 'lost' his ability to eat and lost 15kg in just six weeks. He had made the usual round of doctors but they had been unable to help him. He only contacted me as a last resort. I started by trying to find some event that coincided with the onset of the problem. But after looking in all of the usual places for an emotional upset, shock, or trauma I could find no reason for his condition. It then occurred to me to try something radically different. Using kinesiology (a way of questioning the unconscious through observing the body's responses to questions) I asked if he had been the subject of someone's deliberate ill intention. To my surprise, Kinesiology registered a strong confirming response. With this information we started to use one of the standard energy psychology techniques to eliminate the issue. He was then able to feel the blockage in his body. As the healing process progressed the sensations moved into his hands and fingers. He started shaking them sharply as though trying to throw off something that was clinging to them.

He remembered a girl who wanted to marry him, but whom he had abandoned. She had been sending him messages while he was in the military.

All this was taking place in our garden. I noticed that he was shaking his hands towards a particular bush in the middle of the garden. It suddenly occurred to me to tell him to place his hands on the soil and to allow the earth to absorb whatever energy was disturbing him. This seemed to work since the negative sensations in his hands released. More significantly, he was suddenly overcome by hunger. We offered him food and he finished off everything we placed before him! It turned out that a woman who had been pursuing him for some time, but whom he didn't particularly like, had had to be told that he was not interested in her. It was after this that his problems with eating started. I sensed that the sudden occurrence of a non-human entity attachment on an otherwise healthy young man was due to an act of deliberate ill will - in other words, a spell. The client was delighted with the outcome and wrote a couple of times to thank me for helping him. But for me this successful intervention was about to take an unexpected, and highly unpleasant, turn. The next day I was walking Peanut, my cocker spaniel, in the garden. I had just been thinking to myself how fit and healthy he was for his age, when, as he trotted past the bush I mentioned earlier, he yelped and fell. He couldn't walk – all of the movement in his back legs had been lost and he could only drag himself along with his front legs. Thanks to the dedication and commitment of our vet we were able to help him recover the use of his back legs after three days of treatment. Thankfully he made a full recovery but my shock at this turn of events made me promise myself to never again get involved in cases where ill intention or 'spells' were involved. From now on I would try to send such cases to people who were better equipped to deal with them."

Conclusions

Just because we use traditional words (like 'spirit', 'ghost', 'demon', 'Djinn', 'angel', 'deity', or even the more neutral 'entity') to characterize an anomalous experience does not mean that we are committed to a 'supernatural', in the sense of 'lacking any material base', view of reality. From my own point of view, if a phenomenon can be reasonably categorized as involving a 'spirit' or 'entity' (like the 'ghost' stories and the entity of Edith Turner's healing dance) then I assume that its material basis, like the 96% of the universe that is made of dark energy and dark matter, simply falls outside our usual sensory range and existing technical capabilities. The existence or otherwise of such entities may make for an interesting debate. But when, in the course of routine healing work, you are confronted by phenomena so strongly suggestive of external agency, the main concern is not which theory best accounts for them but how to alleviate people's suffering in a safe and effective way.

At the center of this issue is a critical question, what is the status of the entities that stand at the heart of these phenomena? The concept of unseen entities leaves most of us with a distinct sense of unease. Not so much about the possibility of their existence, a creepy enough idea for sure. Rather, the unease of appearing, to oneself as well as to others, as superstitious, unscientific and, perhaps, a little gullible. The facts themselves seem to exist in a far more complex space than most theories are able to encompass.

Our context is one of healing and in particular, energy healing. All of the cases that we have reviewed so far point towards the fact that our day to day awareness offers only a narrow and partial vantage point from which to survey the broader reality. At the end of the day what we call 'reality' is as much a construction of our perception, and therefore as much 'in our heads', as it is 'out there'.

When we shift, or experience a shift, of awareness the dynamic range of our experience also changes, sometimes radically. When this happens, and depending upon how radical a shift we have made, reality can become unrecognizable from the point of view of consensual reality. Is this reality more or less real than that of our daily lives? From the perspective of the healer it doesn't matter. What does matter is the healing process. The dedicated healer follows their heart, empathy guides them to the heart of the matter. The fact that they can achieve success rates of anything up to or over 90% by facilitating a client's own use of purely natural (non-pharmacological) approaches is itself proof of the validity of their perceptions.

Phenomena occurring at the very edges of human experience are radically 'underdetermined', we simply have too little information to frame a proper understanding of them. The truth, Wilde remarked, is seldom plain and never simple and this is certainly true of anomalous phenomena. Whilst there are many aspects that defy rational understanding, nevertheless the evidence for their validity is too strong for us to dismiss. As a result we need to extend our cognitive model by integrating far more factors than we usually allow for. Jacques Vallee, a prominent researcher of anomalous phenomena, has proposed a model for their interpretation that employs six simultaneous dimensions or 'layers of interpretation'[13]. The layers are:

- Physical: displays a physical presence consistent with other physical objects (eg. passes in front of or behind other objects, reflects light, heat and so on)
- Anti-physical: displays a physical presence inconsistent with those of other physical objects (eg. abruptly appears or disappears, passes through other physical objects)
- Psychological: triggers emotional responses (fear, surprise, altered states of consciousness) and confounds our attempts at sensemaking
- Physiological: leaves distinct traces that are not attributable to natural causes
- Psychic: is associated with classical psychic phenomena such as telepathic communication and out of body experiences
- Cultural: plays into our existing narratives and counter-narratives about what is and is not possible

The world of the energy healer occupies a liminal zone 'betwixt and between' where anomalous phenomena become the new norm. The model of reality that evolves in an attempt to understand these phenomena is of a complex, multilayered, multidimensional space inhabited by many orders of being. Each of us can make these worlds more transparent by undertaking the transformation of our own psycho-energetic being. We will cover this topic in the next chapter.

Notes

1. Wolf, AP. 'Gods, ghosts, and ancestors' in 'Religion and ritual in Chinese society' (ed.) (1974) Wolf, AP. 131–182, 356–357

2. Turner, E. (1992) Experiencing Ritual: A New Interpretation of African Healing p.149

3. Turner, E. 'The Reality of Spirits' Shamanism, Spring/Summer 1997 Vol.10, No.1

4. Sogyal Rinpoche (1992) The Tibetan Book of Living and Dying

5. Sagan, S. (1994) Entity Possession: Freeing the Energy-body of Negative Influences

6. Greenwood, MT. ibid

7. Fiore, E. (1987) The Unquiet Dead: A Psychologist Treats Spirit Possession.

8. Sanderson, Dr. A. 'The Case for Spirit Release' Royal College of Psychiatry, Spirituality Special Interest Group (SIG) Resources.

9. Modi, Dr. S. (1998) Remarkable Healings: A Psychiatrist Discovers Unsuspected Roots of Mental and Physical Illness

10. Baldwin, WJ. & Fiore, E. (1995) Spirit Releasement Therapy: A Technique Manual.

11. Also 'Guei' or 'Kuei'

12. Greenwood, MT. 'Possession' *Medical Acupuncture, Volume 20, Number 1, 2008*

13. Vallee, JF. & Davis, EW *'Incommensurability, Orthodoxy and the Physics of High Strangeness: A 6-layer Model for Anomalous Phenomena'* "Science, Religion and Consciousness" *at the University Fernando Pessoa, Porto (Portugal) 24 October 2003.*

Chapter 7

Healing through Spirit

Peak Experiences

The idea of 'healing through spirit' can be interpreted in two different ways. We can think of it in terms of the healing that occurs as a result of having a spiritual experience. Alternatively, we can think of it as the healing that arises from the intercession of spiritual forces. We will cover both of these interpretations in the course of this chapter. Healing as a result of spiritual experience can manifest on many different levels: physically, emotionally, mentally or spiritually. Because of the profound nature of the such experiences, it is not easy to conceptualize them let alone put them into words as the following account, supplied by a close friend, illustrates.

"One day I was sitting in the kitchen. It was sometime around ten in the morning. My son was about 6 months old then. The house was quiet and we were alone, taking in some quiet time together. He was sitting on my lap, making sounds that babies make and I leaned back against the wall, gazing out at the sea. Then something happened. For maybe what was a second if that, every boundary disappeared. There was no me, no son, no kitchen, no building, no sea, no sky. Everything blended together and the only way I can describe this is a vast nothingness with everything inside. There was nothing as I know but there was everything all at once. It was a second of utter peace, contentment and of being 'whole' yet being nothing at the same time. And then it was gone. Like an accordion closing, just as suddenly as they had disappeared all the boundaries fell back in. I was back in the kitchen, my son was on my lap, the sea was out there. Try as hard as I could, I was not able to bring back that feeling again. I have never had the joy of that moment again and I have a feeling that I'm not supposed to. That moment was there to open a door for me. At the time, I wasn't able to see that door. Many years later, I understand what I was taught that day. In fact it was probably something beyond teaching ... it was an experience, permission to see what it was really all about. I don't understand why I was allowed to see beyond that door but I am thankful for it."

Reading this account we have the distinctive sense of someone having a highly significant experience, but one which remains inexpressible. They can report what they experienced to a certain degree, but its deeper significance and impact somehow eludes us. We are left to ponder what the lesson was, why the experience was so uplifting and in what respect it could be considered a healing experience.

Fresh understanding as to why such experiences are so significant has emerged from recent clinical practice. Psilocybin, the psychoactive ingredient found in certain 'magic mushrooms', has been given to terminally ill patients suffering from depression and end of life anxiety. The subjects described how this drug allowed them to experience a shift from ego centered awareness towards a much larger egoless state of consciousness in which their personal problems vanished and they could empathically review their lives and relationships. One of the researchers, Dr. Charles S. Grob, has described how,

> "Under the influence of hallucinogens individuals transcend their primary identification with their bodies and experience ego-free states before the time of their actual physical demise, and return with a new perspective and profound acceptance of the life constant: change."[1]

This description is also a good description of the typical outcome of much spiritual experience. Such experiences are also called 'peak experiences', a term coined by the psychologist and one of the founders of the Transpersonal Movement in psychology, Abraham Maslow[2].

One of our recurrent themes has been the breadth of the average person's exposure to prescient, anomalous or otherworldly experiences. Peak experiences are no different. Even in secularized societies, such as the UK, surveys concerning people's spiritual experience reveals a surprisingly widespread sense of spirituality. When asked questions such as, "Have you ever felt as though you were very close to a powerful spiritual force that seemed to lift you out of yourself?", close to three quarters of people answered affirmatively[3]. Drawing on the work of the pioneering psychologist, William James[4], and the educator, Frederick Happold[5], Douglas Shrader[6] has proposed a useful summary of some of the key characteristics of such experiences:

Ineffability - it is difficult to do justice to the experience in ordinary language.

Noetic quality - provides insights or understanding beyond those accessible to rational thought.

Transiency - typically lasts for a relatively brief period of time.

Passivity - although these experiences can be facilitated through processes of profound inner cultivation, their occurrence is normally outside of a person's control.

Unity of opposites - awareness of the Oneness of everything.

Timelessness - time stops, there is no sense of duration.

Emptiness of self realization that the phenomenal ego is not the real I, encounter with a deeper sense of selfhood.

Three significant features of peak experiences are overlooked in these points. Firstly, peak experiences are often accompanied by the experience of a pure, ecstatic joy and love for all existence. Secondly, not all peak experiences are transient. It is possible, with suitable yogic accomplishment, to stabilize a peak experiences or even gain sufficient mastery to attain one at will. Thirdly, even transient peak experiences have lasting effects on our worldview, way of life and ethical outlook. Peak experiences are dramatic and compelling. But their real value lies in effecting an ethical shift in the quality of our understanding, depth of compassion and behavior.

Whilst peak experiences are much more common in the overall population than we might expect, in terms of most people's day to day experience they remain rare, spontaneous, wholly unexpected, and extremely transient. The instant we recognize that we are having such an experience, our awareness 'snaps back' to its habitual egocentered focus. If such states are to become anything more than transient phenomena, clearly something more is required. Classically this has involved parallel activity in three main areas:

- Purification of the psycho-physical organism. This involves both the integration of outstanding mental and emotional issues and the detoxification of the physical body. In some systems (such as the many forms of spiritual yoga) it also covers the opening of the energy channels and the cultivation (refinement and expansion) of life-energy.

- Training the mind through systematic meditative and contemplative practice. This allows the mind to become accustomed to remaining in a state of present moment, non-judgmental awareness. It also develops the capacity to recognize higher states as they unfold without becoming distracted by them.

- Adopting a practical, service based orientation to life. Apart from the inherent merits of such activities, they serve to maintain an appropriate relationship with reality. The discipline of serving helps to strengthen our capacity for empathy and compassionate action.

The experience of higher states is not the 'property' or 'accomplishment' of the ego. The ego will inevitably try to appropriate all spiritual realizations as its own accomplishment. In fact the logic of spiritual states works the other way around. Spiritual realization is the experience that arises when the ego finally gets out of the way. The world's many spiritual traditions contain numerous examples of people who have stabilized their awareness at these higher levels. Drawing upon these rich sources we see that the progress towards realization possesses a definite structure both in terms of the stages and types of experience encountered.

The Stages of the Path

Based on her own experience and the comparison of accounts in classic works of mysticism, the poet and mystic Evelyn Underhill proposed a five step process that characterizes the movement of our awareness towards the experience of higher states[7]. When stripped of their theological language, we arrive at the following generic stages on the path.

Awakening. This often includes such existential changes as becoming disenchanted with the limitations of one's life, becoming aware of or suspecting the existence of a higher order of reality and developing the aspiration to work towards it. This realization can arise in many different ways. Most of us are immersed in the intensity and demands of day to day living. And yet, from time to time, we experience the feeling that there must be much more to life. We may even feel that this life is just a stage in a much larger process, the outlines of which we can barely sense. Others may feel completely disillusioned with all aspects of life and be hungry for some higher purpose or meaning. However the process is triggered, an active quest for greater meaning and sense of purpose and understanding is embarked upon.

Purgation. Purgation involves a progressive awareness of one's imperfections, the growth of the motivation necessary for self-improvement and the determination to master the techniques and practices necessary to achieve this. For many people this is as far as they are able to get since the effective use of the available techniques and practices demands self-discipline, commitment, and systematic practice. They also require a degree of external supervision. Identifying and then working on our most sensitive issues is never easy, and there are seemingly an infinite number of distractions that allow us to avoid doing so. With supervision and the choice of the most appropriate techniques the chances of success can be greatly increased. Getting rid of your TV and minimizing the time you spend on the internet are essential prerequisites!

Illumination. Prolonged practice leads to episodes of direct awareness of the unitive order underlying all things. These insights might occur quite rarely at first and last for only a short time, but with prolonged practice their frequency and duration increases. Although transitory, these experiences can have a lasting effect.

They tend to broaden our awareness and lead us towards a larger conception of life-purpose within a much broader understanding of reality.

The Dark Night of the Soul. This phrase is taken from a classic 16th century work of mysticism of that name by Saint John of the Cross[8]. Prolonged and disciplined practice leads to the progressive dissolution or relativization of the ego as awareness starts to break free from the habitual attachments that have 'moored' it in relation to everyday life. This is experienced as a process of dissolution or slow death. For this reason it is sometimes called the *Nekyia,* night voyage or, 'dark night of the soul'. In the language of alchemy it corresponds to the *Nigredo* or blackening stage.

Realization or Union. The final stage, realization or union, is comprised of several successive levels or depths. It can manifest itself in many different ways that may be influenced by the symbols and practices of the tradition within which you are practicing. Whilst this model provides a useful framework for thinking about the process of spiritual development, we need to recognize that it is founded on theistic meditative and contemplative practices. The object of practice within theistic traditions is usually described as union with the deity. The Catholic mystic, poet and writer Thomas Merton has described the experience of mystical union,

> "Contemplation goes beyond concepts and apprehends God not as a separate object but as the Reality within our reality, the Being within our being, the life of our life."[9]

Other traditions, especially non-theistic ones, may conceptualize the process in more abstract terms, as the following extract from a classical Taoist text shows,

> "One bright ray of light hovers over the Dharma universe. When both are forgotten, stillness is numinous and empty. In the void of the great expanse, the celestial mind shines. The waters of the ocean are clear and the moon is reflected in

the deep lake. When there is no birth there will be no death. Nothing leaves and nothing comes."[10]

It is not easy to make comparisons between such diverse experiences, even though we suspect that they are pointing to the same underlying realization. They are separated by significant historical and cultural differences. Each is expressed in its own traditional language and symbolism. Nevertheless, many people feel that, at some deeper level, humanity accesses a common core of spiritual experience and realization. A useful model that we can use to explore this insight has been proposed by professor of religion, Robert Forman. His model differentiates three progressively deeper levels of realization: the Pure Consciousness Event, the Dualistic Mystical State and the Unitive Mystical State[11].

a) The Pure Consciousness Event (PCE): is a wakeful but content-less (non-intentional) experience. Remaining awake and alert whilst neither thinking nor acting and emerging with the clear sense of having had "an unbroken continuity of experience".

b) Dualistic Mystical State (DMS): being in touch with our own deepest awareness, experienced as silence, while remaining fully conscious of the external world.

c) Unitive Mystical State (UMS): experiencing one's awareness as inseparable from the totality of all things, expansive and field-like.

The Unitive Mystical State marks the outer limits or horizon of human awareness. Attempts to describe it are often marked by contradiction and paradox. A typical example being the classical Taoist saying, "The Tao that can be spoken is not the eternal Tao"[12]. Despite the ineffability of these experiences we do encounter some striking commonalities that transcend time and culture. The experience of the 17th century Welsh mystic, Henry Vaughan, bears direct comparison with that of Maria Sabina, a 20th century Mexican shaman. The vision that they are describing recurs often enough, and with more or less the same quality and imagery, for it to be called 'The Vision of the Machinery of the Universe':

> "I saw Eternity the other night, Like a great ring of pure and endless light, All calm, as it was bright; And round beneath it, Time in hours, days, years, Driv'n by the spheres Like a vast shadow mov'd; in which the world And all her train were hurl'd".[13]

> "you see our past and our future, which are there together as a thing already achieved, already happened... I knew and saw God: an immense clock that ticks, the spheres that go slowly around, and inside the stars, the earth, the entire universe, the day, the night"[14]

Peak experiences, such as these, affect us on many different levels. Mentally they affirm the insight that all sentient life is connected at some deeper level of being. Emotionally they provide the confidence that arises from knowing that we endure through many different lives. Physically they are accompanied by feelings of ecstatic bliss traceable to shifts in our inner energy. Over the longer term they free us from the self-obsession, fear and futility of ego-centered awareness. But even taking all of these factors into account we are still left with the question, what is it that makes these experiences so culturally significant?

The Evolutionary Unfolding of Consciousness

*"Evolution is a light illuminating all facts, a
curve that all lines must follow."*

Teilhard de Chardin

Through cases involving psychic knowing, merged identities, past lives, family and ancestral healing we have seen how all sentient life is immersed in a vast, timeless 'web of life'. We have called the portion of this web common to experiences of healing and personal transformation as The Healing Field. It is constituted of information and a degree of harmony/disharmony that, experienced through the lens of human awareness, renders positive and negative emotional affects, personal meaning and ethical values.

The lives of individuals, families and all sentient life forms are influenced by, and in turn influence, this multilayered field of consciousness. It has been variously called the collective unconscious (CG Jung), the 'Morphic Field' (Rupert Sheldrake), the Akashic or 'Afield' (Ervin Laszlo) and 'The Knowing Field' (Albrecht Mahr).

In the context of family constellations we saw how patterns of negative affect, coded in the field through trauma and injustice, create patterns of disharmony that affect the health and well-being of subsequent generations. We also saw how these patterns can be decoded, brought into the light of day through symbolic re-enactment, and then recoded to eliminate their negativity. This process, one of 'ethical reharmonization', provides us with a context to understand the spiritual value of peak experiences. They are important because they recode patterns of negative affect and provide a more compassionate and stable basis for future action. In short, meditative and peak experiences facilitate the co-creation of reality from a broader, more compassionate perspective.

At the very heart of most of the spiritual paths for which the five stage model is relevant we find the mastery of certain meditative practices. Meditation is not so much one single technique as the generic name for a range of loosely related techniques and practices.

The Range of Meditative Practices

Of his time spent in silent retreat in a monastery, the famous travel writer Patrick Leigh Fermor has written,

"in the seclusion … the troubled waters of the mind grow still and clear, and much that is hidden away and all that clouds it floats to the surface and can be skimmed away; and after a time one reaches a state of peace that is un-thought of in the ordinary world."[15]

Whilst the actual practice of meditation means different things to different people, most of us will probably agree that it should lead to the kind of inner peace and quiet described above. In practical terms meditation covers a wide range of techniques and practices. Some of these have been evolved over many thousands of years within different traditions and are designed to achieve specific objectives. Within this vast range of practices we can discern, at least, five basic patterns of meditative practice:

Mindfulness meditation, which consists in maintaining a state of present moment, non-judgmental awareness. Developing skill with mindfulness is a 'core' discipline in many traditions. Mindfulness has proven mental and physical medical benefits as well as developing the non-attachment that is essential for the manifestation and stabilization of higher states of awareness.

Single pointed meditation, which consists of maintaining focus on a single point. This practice is used to develop concentration.

Compassion meditation, a heart centered meditation that often involves reaching out to all sentient beings and wishing for the alleviation of their suffering.

Contemplation, a form of meditation involving the meditative exploration of a particular topic or question.

Yogic meditation, an advanced practice that involves some combination of meditative stillness, visualization, sound, breathing, posture and energy work.

Yogic meditative practice, along with other forms of excitation, represents an alternative path to spiritual realization that forms the subject matter of the next section.

The Energized Path to Realization

The five stages of spiritual realization provide a useful model for understanding quietist traditions, such as the many forms of monasticism that utilize contemplative and meditative practice. Quietude involves withdrawing from sensory excitation, embracing quiet, solitary conditions and developing a capacity for stilling the mind and entering profound states of inner quiet. This path can be contrasted with the paths of excitation and energized meditation. Both excitation and energized meditation use high levels of inner energy to force the rapid expansion of awareness. The paths of quietude, excitation and energized meditation all ultimately 'meet' at the highest levels of spiritual realization the unitive mystical state (see diagram below).

Excitation may involve any combination of music, dance, singing, chanting, energized breathing as well as the use of powerful, mind expanding substances or entheogens. These practices constitute a form of rapid induction capable of quickly raising the powerful life-energy (called kundalini) situated at the base of the spine. They are often encountered in aboriginal ritual, for example, the Healing Dance of the Kalahari Kung people.

The extent to which everyone in the community gets involved in the Healing Dance does much to offset the strangeness that inevitably surrounds these practices. The Healing Dance starts during daytime with women sitting in a group and singing, often with their children, whilst accompanying themselves by clapping. The men join in by commencing a stamping dance around the women. This singing and dancing continues for many hours far into the night. As it progresses the rhythm of the dancing intensifies. The dance activates the inner energy of the dancers – called num – located (exactly like its yogic equivalent, Kundalini) in the stomach and base of the spine,

> "Num, this primary force in the Kung's universe of experience, is at its strongest in the healing dance.... The num in the healer must be activated for it to become a healing energy. The Kung say the num must 'gam' or rise up. The singing of songs helps awaken the num and awaken the healer's heart ... The Kung feel that their hearts must awaken or open before they attempt to heal."[16]

As the singing and dancing proceeds the quality of the energy intensifies. Some people drop out as the energy becomes too intense for them to handle. At a certain point the energy 'boils' and rises up the spine to give rise to a greatly expanded state of awareness called 'kia'. In this state the healers can 'see' illnesses inside other people's bodies, pull the illnesses out, remote view over great distances and commune with spirits and gods.

The healing that takes place has three main aspects: 'seeing' the underlying causes of mental and physical problems. 'Pulling out' the illness, depicted as arrows piercing the ill person, either by using the hands or by absorbing the illness into the healer's own body and then expelling it. Interceding with the gods on the behalf of the sick person and resisting any spirits or ghosts sent to take the sick person 'away'. The practices of the *Kung* healers are paralleled by traditional shaman the world over as well as by certain energy healers. You may recall my own experience with this form of healing described in the first pages of this book.

Diagram V: The Paths of Quietude & Excitation

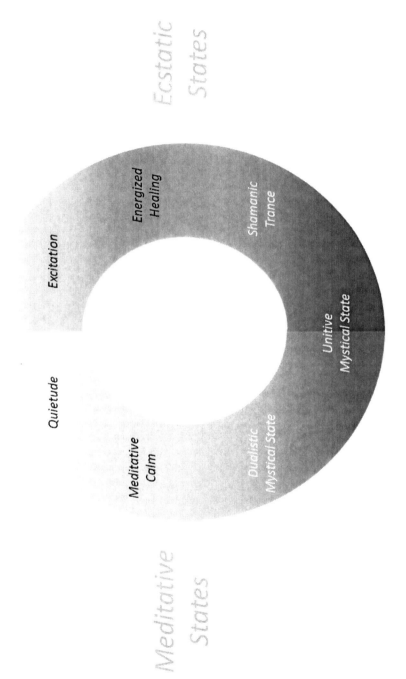

The traditional practices of kundalini yoga and Qi Gung describe similar transmutations of inner energy, experienced as extreme internal heat. These Eastern disciplines are usually practiced on a daily basis for many years. Compared to this the raising of kundalini energy during the Healing Dance occurs in just several hours. It is this that accounts for the difficulty, discomfort and danger experienced by the participants,

> "The training is difficult. Not everyone can stand the excruciating pain of boiling num, said to be "hot and painful, just like fire". It makes one cry and writhe in agony. Part of the pain comes from facing one's own death. To heal one must die and be reborn ... The terror of kia remains despite years of healing, and accepting this recurrent death is the core of the healer's training."[17]

From accounts like this it is clear that the path of excitation is not for everyone. The alternative path of energized meditation is typical of the many schools of Indo-Tibetan and Chinese yoga. These traditions utilize a sophisticated combination of practices including meditation, posture, diet, breathing and visualization combined with quietude to realize the high levels of inner energy that in turn speed the processes of inner purification and the refinement. Progress can be accelerated by receiving direct energy transfers from a master practitioner. Such energy transfers can be delivered with different levels of strength up to and including initiations that trigger peak experiences. It is then up to the practitioner to establish a physical, emotional and psycho-spiritual foundation capable of stabilizing their awareness at these higher levels.

Within the traditions of spiritual yoga the stabilization of enlightened realization is facilitated by the manipulation of the fundamental energies that support and sustain relative awareness. Using techniques such as breath suspension (Kevala Kumbhaka) these fundamental energetic supports are progressively withdrawn into the central energy channel (the Sushumna) where they 'collapse' upon themselves giving rise to enlightened awareness[18].

This collapse parallels the processes that occur naturally at death. It is, perhaps for this reason that the approach of spiritual realization can be accompanied by such feelings of dread. Ultimately, all paths converge in a common experience of spiritual unity. Irrespective of the techniques used, the structure of the experience will often exhibit four distinct stages:

- Firstly, there is a growing dissolution of our sense of selfhood. This is usually accompanied by feelings of fear and dread, as though dying to this world. In mystical tradition this stage is called the 'dark night of the soul'.

- Secondly, at the deepest point of this 'collapse' of our sense of biographical selfhood there is a sudden ecstatic expansion of awareness where all sense of time and place are lost as everything is absorbed into unity.

- Thirdly, coming down from the ecstasy of union there will be prolonged period of inner stillness and peace.

- Fourthly, in the days and weeks that follow there will be a gradual resumption of one's habitual connections with reality though in a uniquely 'relativized' way they will simply fail to hold the same addictive and compulsive attraction that they once had.

The following account of an experience of kundalini rising illustrates many of these points,

"I sat on a low hill, a still, moonlit swathe of grass ringed by distant trees that stood like a dark enclosure, containing reality. My mood plunged with a receding tide of vitality, down, down. I ventured towards the gates of hell, a great gaping darkness, the fear of total engulfment. Patience is the only virtue in such situations, waiting it out and waiting, like an expectant surfer, for the next wave to come. Sure enough it starts to stir, deep in the base of the spine, at first, just the faintest of vibrations that signals my trains a comin'. The vibrations grow. They grow and expand with the joy of life itself. And then it comes. Unstoppable, pure liquid fire surges up my spine, ecstasy of life, consciousness expands to the four quarters. Bliss beyond bliss. I am all and all is in me. I surf the tides of existence. There is nothing to fear, we always were and always will be. Hours later I return to earth. For days afterwards I am at peace and harmony with all of life. I see and feel the beauty of every living thing. As the days pass, I come down. Things start, once more, to bother me. I become a burden to myself. Small irritations trouble me, I doubt everything, fear the future and regret the loss of time once more, as though time were finite But now I can comfort myself. I know and can say - this is all illusion."

This overall process is consistent enough to allow us to depict its main contours (diagram below). The direct paths of excitation and energized meditation are not for everyone. There are significant risks involved in any attempt to force the pace of spiritual development. The dangers are real and take a number of forms. Collectively they are known as 'spiritual emergencies'.

Diagram VI: The Dynamics of Spiritual Experience

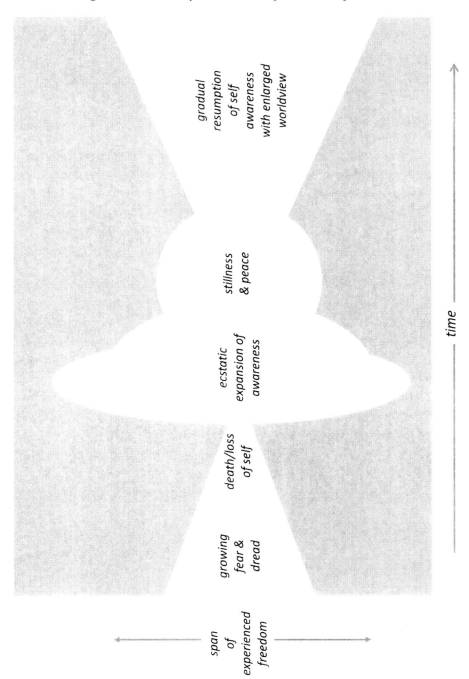

span of experienced freedom

growing fear & dread

death/loss of self

ecstatic expansion of awareness

stillness & peace

gradual resumption of self awareness with enlarged worldview

time

Spiritual Emergencies

Stanislav Grof, a psychiatrist and one of the founders of the transpersonal movement in psychology, noted the Western tendency to diagnose shifts in our awareness as psychopathological problems, rather than as opportunities for personal growth and transformation,

> "There exist spontaneous non-ordinary states that would in the west be seen and treated as psychosis, treated mostly by suppressive medication. But … they should really be treated as crises of transformation, or crises of spiritual opening. … If properly understood and .. supported, they are actually conducive to healing and transformation."[19]

By and large, modern industrial and post-industrial societies lack the kinds of informal, knowledgeable, community based networks that are supportive of such healing and transformation. The preferred approach to the mass anxiety faced in these societies is to engage in their wholesale suppression using a broad range of tranquilizers and anti-depressants. Few people are well equipped or supported to engage in profound personal or spiritual transformation. For this reason we should not overlook the very real dangers associated with certain practices used to accelerate such changes. This is especially true of the states induced by some of the more extreme practices encountered during shamanic initiation or with the more extreme and/or intense forms of meditation and yoga – especially, kundalini yoga.

People undertaking intensive meditative and yogic practices can, as a result of the powerful processes used to purify the psycho-physical organism, experience the activation of latent illnesses or the traces of past illnesses as they are flushed from the body. People with a history of mental illness, suffering from unresolved emotional issues or under high levels of stress in their day to day life may experience an intensification of these conditions. If pushed too far, this intensification may become too overwhelming for them to be integrated and lead to a 'psychic blowout' – a phrase used to describe the experience of becoming overwhelmed and no longer able to continue with any practice or cope with reality itself.

The adage about making haste slowly applies to all forms of inner work and spiritual development. Perhaps the most important lesson is not to engage in intensive practices, whether it's running a marathon or meditating continuously for a number of days, without first building up your capacity to a level approximating what you are planning to undertake. Following this one simple rule would save many people all manner of mental, physical and emotional disturbances. Even for a regular, daily meditator a week long intensive is going to be, well, very intense. In this context it is useful to look at the mixture of healing and distress experienced by a regular meditator during a meditation intensive[20].

The first day involved intense physical discomfort that arose from maintaining a meditative position for far longer periods than he was used to. Through the next few days the meditator experienced increasingly deeper levels of peace and a broadening quality of awareness until by day 5 he was able to say, "I experienced bliss". But by day 6 he was feeling troubled, "The peace and calm of previous days began to elude me. Thoughts and feelings of conceit, self-consciousness, and judgment surfaced frequently. During a group debriefing session on the final day he reported, "I was overcome by emotion as I tried to speak ... My eyes welled up with tears, I felt emotionally raw." In conclusion he stated, "Overall, I found the experience healing, self-expanding, calming, rejuvenating, and deeply transpersonal. I experienced stillness, quiet, and self-observation at levels never before encountered." It is just such an opportunity, to experience a profound shift in our awareness that we can take back into our everyday lives and use to improve how we live and interact with others, that explains why the path of meditative stillness is so attractive to so many people.

Cases of spiritual emergency demonstrate the extent to which our 'normal' day to day awareness is blind to our deeper mental, physical, emotional and energetic condition. This is one measure of our self-alienation. Intense quietude merely forces us to confront who we really are and what our true condition and posture in life is. In addition to meditative stillness we can utilize a whole range of techniques to cleanse, purify and cultivate our inner energy in order to speed up and stabilize the processes of transformation. The downside of such practices is an appreciable increase in the risk of mental, physical and emotional destabilization.

Given the many difficulties, the likelihood of failure, and the very real dangers associated with the path of energized meditation, why, you might well ask, would anyone be bothered to undertake such a journey? There is no easy answer. But I suspect that it emerges from a deep impulse to transcend the limitations of our present condition by moving towards some 'higher ground' with respect to our humanity and to fully realize a hidden – but deeply felt – potential within ourselves, an upward moving and expansive impulse inherent in all sentient beings. In short, it is an evolutionary imperative.

Because of the difficulties of attempting a solo ascent of the mystical path, millennia old traditions have emerged that integrate guidance and direct initiation from an ascending scale of beings. These are traditionally called fully realized teachers, ascended masters, enlightened beings, angels and, ultimately, gods and demi-gods. One form in which this help materializes is by way of a transmission of energy to the aspirant that triggers varying degrees of peak experience. This process corresponds to the second interpretation that we can give to the phrase 'healing through spirit'. Earlier, in the context of healing on extended planes of existence, we saw that other forms of awareness of varying degrees of sentience also interact with us via the morphic fields of shared consciousness. No account of the spiritual path, and its effects on the evolution of the fields of sentient consciousness, would be complete without considering the higher order beings that interact with us via the morphic fields of shared consciousness.

The Transmission of Energy

*"Be watchful — the grace of God appears suddenly.
It comes without warning to an open heart."*

Rumi

Many approaches to spiritual development are mediated through a personal connection with higher order beings. Short of personal experience, this idea will strike most people as extremely dubious if not highly unlikely. One of the problems is that the experiences that underpin these ideas are extremely rare, fall entirely outside mainstream thinking and only occur to people who are dedicated to and practicing a specific spiritual path. This makes instances of such 'contact' private and worthy of our respect. But wider indications of their validity do sometimes occur, as the following account illustrates,

"Many years ago I reluctantly accompanied my partner to a 'New Age' event. It was a seminar by Tom Kenyon, a popular New Age figure. At the time I had no idea who he was nor did I have any information about him. In the seminar Tom claimed that he had been contacted during his meditative practice by a group of intergalactic, interdimensional beings he called the Hathors (a name derived from the ancient Egyptian fertility goddess). He stated that these beings exist at a very much higher vibrational rate than ourselves and our day to day reality. During the event Tom sought to connect the audience with these beings through his sacred vocal music. This music is inspired by the Hathors and channeled by Tom. As Tom sang I distinctly 'saw', that's to say 'psychically registered', the presence of many tall columns of light around the stage. These columns seemed to move out and through the audience. One of them appeared to come straight towards and pass through me. Much later on, during a question and answer session, a member of the audience asked Tom what these beings looked like. You can imagine my surprise when he described them as 'tall columns of light'.

The role of higher order beings is to facilitate the transmission of purifying energies and teachings. Such transmissions form an integral part of all higher rites of spiritual initiation. These rites are quite unlike the 'rites of passage' that effect changes in a person's social status (such as the transition from childhood to adulthood). Instead, the rites of spiritual initiation are voluntary, typically undertaken by only a small percentage of people and may, depending upon their depth and profundity, involve intensive preparation and purification. They often require the aspirant to take binding vows of secrecy, to abstain from certain behaviors and activities and to strive to perform certain practices and act in charitable and ethical ways. Finally, they may involve vows of secrecy regarding the initiation process and what is experienced during it. Initiates may form a social group that holds its own private meetings, engages in communal acts of charity and represents itself as a cohesive force for good in society at large.

One of the most accessible and widely known forms of such initiation is the worldwide practice of Usui Reiki. Reiki is an initiatory, easy to use and highly effective form of hands-on energy healing. Worldwide all Usui Reiki practitioners can trace their 'lineage' through initiatic transmission from Reiki teacher to Reiki teacher, all the way back to Mikao Usui (1875-1923). Usui was a Tendai Buddhist with an interest in the cultivation of inner energy. He appears to have 'elaborated' the practice of Reiki from a range of pre-existing elements and traditions, but the energy itself came to him spontaneously during a meditation. It is the continuity in teacher to teacher transmission that distinguishes authentic Usui Reiki from the many other traditions of hands-on healing therapy that exist today. Some of these are extremely ancient, such as those practiced within the disciplines of Qi Gung or yoga. Across central Asia and into the Middle East a range of traditional hands-on healing techniques are known and practiced. Many of these are maintained within ancestral lineages connected to people who were recognized for their spirituality and psychic talents. Other traditions, such as bioenergy, constitute a recognized form of medicine in some societies. Still others are of very recent origin, having sprung up over the last 10 years or so. Some of these later forms of hands-on healing describe themselves as 'reiki' though it would be more accurate to describe them as 'reiki-like' since they have no connection with Usui Reiki and draw upon sources of energy unique to their own tradition.

Reiki's effectiveness is such that it is slowly gaining institutional acceptance both as a research subject and as a component of conventional medical treatment[21]. Reiki is now available in some 15% of US hospitals. This form of 'integrated medicine' has proved to be highly popular and has become the preferred patient care model in most of the world's leading hospitals. In a recent survey it was found that 60% of the top 25 US hospitals have Reiki programs in place. These include both outside Reiki Professionals providing services at a hospital as well as nursing staff trained in providing Reiki as an adjunct or complementary therapy. Of the hospitals that do not have Reiki programs in place, 50% are open to offering Reiki in the future.

One of the advantages of Reiki is that it is a thoroughly secular practice. It is not necessary to 'believe in' Reiki, or anything else for that matter, in order to either provide or receive effective Reiki treatment. Although people have inevitably tended to embed Reiki within their own belief systems, Reiki itself remains independent of any beliefs. Reiki is compatible with all belief systems – or none.

There would be no point in addressing any of these issues if there was not a clear consensus concerning Reiki's effectiveness amongst its millions of practitioners and recipients worldwide. Whether being used to support greater relaxation or to allay acute physical pain, Reiki can be aptly described as a 'universal panacea'. But what kind of 'energy' is it, where does it 'come from', what's its source and how does it work to promote universal health and healing? The answer is, we simply don't know. What is clear, however, is that the effectiveness of Reiki is not a result of the Placebo Effect[22]. You will recall the remarkable case of Gulcan's aged mother who healed herself of an otherwise intractable condition whilst under medical supervision so that her improvement was monitored by a medical specialist who went on to become a Reiki practitioner himself!

The world of Reiki is rich in accounts of remarkable healing. Amongst dedicated Reiki practitioners the explanation is simple. Reiki is a spiritually directed healing energy. Spiritually directed means just that, though the nature of the spiritual direction remains obscure. Modernity and its positivist 'what you see is all there is' worldview refutes the idea of higher order beings even though they have been attested in every culture from time immemorial. Although we think of such beings as 'supernatural', that is, as lacking a material basis, all it really means is that their material basis, like the 96% of the universe made of dark energy and matter, is quite invisible and unknown to us. And yet when we open ourselves to the higher frequencies of love, compassion and healing, 'they', whoever 'they' are, are ready to work with us.

"We have been teaching Reiki for some 15 years. Whenever we 'graduated' a new set of Reiki Teachers we always celebrated the occasion and, inevitably, took photographs of the new graduates and their certificates. On one occasion we took a group photograph of the new graduates in our training room. Gulcan was standing next to them and drew one of the Reiki 'symbols' whilst she called upon the energy to be present with us. This happened just as I was taking the photograph. Something very strange then occurred. I took the photograph using its built-in flash and as I looked through the viewfinder and clicked the camera the flash 'bounced back' straight into my eyes. It was as though I had taken a flash photograph directly into a mirror. I blinked, checked the camera as I thought to myself "that was strange", I had better take that again. I did and the same thing happened. Finally, on the third attempt, the camera took the photograph 'normally'. When we uploaded the pictures to the PC the area around Gulcan, where she had drawn the Reiki 'symbol' in the air, displayed a great circle of light, the inner parts of which had clear 3dimensional properties whilst its outer edges dissipated outwards blurring the surrounding space in front of the group. Several of the group had distinctive 'halos' around their heads. There was no mirror or other reflective surface behind the group to account for the flashback from the camera. Whatever manifested in response to being called was real, not imagined since it had recordable reflective properties. The second photograph had distinct residual effects whilst the third photograph was more or less normal" (see photograph below).

Although, as the quotation from Rumi indicates, transmission can occur spontaneously, as 'divine grace' or 'Baraka', it is more commonly associated with rites of spiritual initiation specifically designed to impart this energy. Such rites can be of varying degrees of complexity. They can be accomplished through a simple gesture, such as touching one of the 'chakras' as in the yogic practice of 'shaktipat'. In the case of Usui Reiki the initiation process is a simple procedure requiring just a few movements that can be comfortably performed in 10 to 20 minutes. The profundity of the resulting experience depends heavily upon the candidate. With proper inner preparation and an open heart, even a simple Reiki initiation can trigger a profound spiritual experience. The following account is from my own initiation into the Usui Reiki second degree,

"During my Usui Reiki second degree initiation I experienced entering a bright light. It was of high intensity but without being in any way harsh or blinding. The sense I had of it was of a higher vibratory state. I could make out very little but I distinctly sensed the presence of a number of figures within the light. I felt as though they surrounded me and embraced me. I was drowned in a sense of shared unity, acceptance and love. I stayed as long as I could and then felt myself slowly falling back to normal awareness. As I returned to myself I was overcome by a great sadness and sense of loss. As though I had fallen from a state of grace – a state of shared and fully realized bliss, back into gross matter. I don't know how long this experience lasted but it must have been for some length of time for when I 'returned' everyone else had finished, and I was left sitting alone."

Photographs taken after a group healing session with Reiki

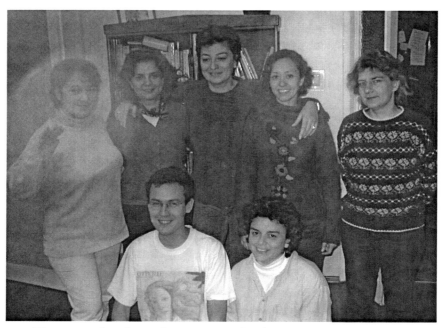

Photograph taken after a group healing session with Reiki

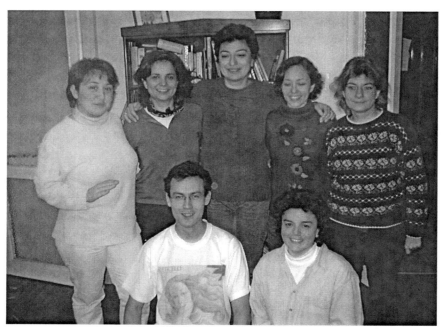

Photograph taken after a group healing
session with Reiki 4 seconds later

In the context of shamanism, the instruction of the shaman is often undertaken by beings connected with his ancestral lineage. Similarly, the rites of higher initiation are frequently associated with the intercession of specific beings who maintain a special relationship with the lineage-holders. These are people who have dedicated their lives to preserving the teachings, rituals and initiation rites. Contemporary examples of such rites are the IndoTibetan rites of the higher yoga tantra, also known as deity yoga. A parallel system, known as Dzogchen, provides a direct initiatory path to the realization of spiritual enlightenment. It is said of this system that it was brought to this planet by a fully realized interdimensional being who took a human incarnation for this specific purpose. The system he taught and provided initiation into is said to be practiced in thirteen other solar systems[23].

As we noted, the initiations themselves serve a variety of purposes. They are undertaken for healing and inner purification; to 'attune' a person or group to a healing energy so that they become empowered to either use or pass on that healing energy in turn; to convey the experience of spiritual illumination or to attune a person or group to an energy source that can then be invoked to support and facilitate the process of inner development.

The highest spiritual initiations involve the direct transmission of energy from higher order beings. Such initiations can be delivered one-to-one or simultaneously to hundreds of thousands of people at a time with no dilution or diminution of effect. Initiations involving thousands of people that trigger intense states of direct spiritual realization are typical of the highest yoga tantra. Similar rites, known generically as 'the Mysteries', were pervasive throughout the ancient world for at least 3,000 years until they were suppressed in the 4th century CE. The main claim made for the importance of these rites was that they were the key to sustaining civilization itself. Speaking of their initiation into the mysteries of Eleusis some thirty years before, a friend of the Roman statesman Cicero wrote,

"nothing is better than those mysteries. For by means of them we have been civilized ... we have learned from them the fundamentals of life and have grasped the basis not only for living with joy but also for dying with a better hope"[24]

"by means of them, we have been civilized"

One of the main claims made for the importance of the Mysteries was that they sustained civilization itself. They were thought of as holding "the entire human race together"[25]. Why this should be so becomes clearer when we consider the role of spiritual initiation rites in the life of a traditional community. One rite in particular is worth considering, that of the Bwiti religion of West Africa. Briefly, the practitioners of Bwiti conduct a rite that reinforces the ties holding their community together, strengthens their relationship with the ancestral spirits and spirits of the natural world and provides a direct experience of the divine. The rite extends over three days, involves the whole community at certain stages and employs a powerful entheogen called Iboga.

The Bwiti initiation rite follows the traditional three stage process that characterizes most 'rites of passage' – separation, liminality and reintegration[26]. The middle stage of the rite is designed to morally 'purify' the candidate in order to prepare them to meet the powerful spirits of the natural world. This is accomplished by triggering a process of recalling all of the significant events of one's life up to that point. The important feature of this recall is that these events are recalled not from the ordinary self-centered perspective, but from the perspective of the people most affected by them. People who have undergone the rite have testified to its powerful impact on their moral outlook. It 'civilizes' the 'raw' components of personality by making us acutely aware of the consequences of our actions on other people.

Regarding sacred initiation rites the view of modern classical scholarship is that, "the gap between … (ourselves) … and the experience of those involved in the real proceedings remains unbridgeable"[27]. But it is only unbridgeable to the extent that we refrain from undergoing the necessary purification and transformation of our own being and fail to seek out contemporary contexts in which valid initiation still confers an experience of the numinous. As we have seen throughout the course of this book, the walls separating the sacred from the profane, the mundane from the numinous are never too distant for us to reach nor too high for us to overcome.

Notes

1. *Psychiatrist Dr. Charles S. Grob quoted in J. Tierney 'Hallucinogens Have Doctors Tuning In Again' New York Times, April 11, 2010*

2. *Maslow, AH. (1964) Religions, Values and Peak Experiences.*

3. *Hay, D. & Hunt, K. (2000) 'Understanding the Spirituality of People Who Don't Go To Church, Final Report of the Adult Spirituality Project' Nottingham: University of Nottingham*

4. *James, W. (1902) The Varieties of Religious Experience Chapters XVI to XVII*

5. *Happold, FC. (1963) Mysticism: A Study and an Anthology*

6. *Shrader, DW. (2008)'The Seven Characteristics of Mystical Experience' Proceedings of the 6th Annual Hawaii International Conference on Arts and Humanities. Honolulu, HI, 2008.*

7. *Underhill, E. (1911) Mysticism: A Study of the Nature and Development of Man's Spiritual Consciousness*

8. *Dark Night of the Soul by St John of the Cross*

9. *Merton, T. (1978) The New Man p.19*

10. *Hui Ming Ching (The Book of Consciousness and Life) Section 8 (trans) Wong, Eva*

11. *Foreman, R. 'What Does Mysticism Have to Teach us About Consciousness?' Journal of Consciousness Studies, Vol. 5, No. 2, 1998, pp. 185–201*

12. *Tao Te Ching, Chapter 1*

13. *Vaughan, H. (1905) The Poems of Henry Vaughan Silurist*

14. *Schultes, RE., Hofmann, A. & Rätsch, C. (1979) Plants of the Gods: Their Sacred, Healing and Hallucinogenic Powers*

15. *Fermor, PL. (1957) A Time to Keep Silence*

16. Katz, R. (1982) *Boiling Energy: community healing among the Kalahari Kung*

17. Katz, R. 'The Painful Ecstasy of Healing' in Goleman, D. & Davidson, RJ., (eds.) (1979) 'Consciousness: Brain, States of Awareness and Mysticism' pp. 166-169

18. Geshe Lhundub Sopa 'The Subtle Body in Tantric Buddhism' in 'The Wheel of Time: the Kalachakra in Context' (ed.) Simon, B. p.144

19. Interview with Stanislav Grof

20. Johnson, CV. 'Reflections on a Silent Meditation Retreat: A Beginner's Perspective' *International Journal of Transpersonal Studies*, 28, 2009, pp. 134-138

21. Herron-Marx, S., et al. 'A systematic review of the use of Reiki in health care' *Alternative and Complementary Therapies.* 2008, 14(1): 37-42

22. Some of the evidence for its effectiveness has been made available from studies undertaken at Hartford Hospital: http://www.harthosp.org/integrativemed/default.aspx

23. Norbu, N. (1986) *The Crystal and the Way of Light: Sutra, Tantra and Dzogchen* p.13

24. Cicero, *On the Laws*, 2.14.36

25. Kerenyi, C. (1967) *Eleusis: Archetypal Image of Mother and Daughter* p. 11-12 citing a letter of Zosimos

26. Van Gennep, A. (1909) *The Rites of Passage*

27. Burkert, W. (1987) 'Ancient Mystery Cults' p.90-91

Chapter 8

Conclusions

What have these experiences shown us?

Most of us think that what we see is all there is. Yet there is ample evidence that what we see is only a tiny fraction of what there is. Our day to day awareness is like a torch that illuminates only a small circle of light in the surrounding darkness. The vast bulk of reality remains invisible to us. It vibrates at frequencies beyond the range of normal perception, much like the 96% of the universe that is comprised of dark matter and dark energy about which we know nothing whatsoever. Since time immemorial people have engaged in practices that allow them to shift their awareness to take in more of the hidden reality around them. Such practices have formed an integral part of every human culture from the earliest times to the present day. The broader view they reveal is one in which we are able to shift our awareness within many different fields of consciousness. As we do so what we experience, what we think of as 'reality', bends and flexes to accommodate our different perspectives. The fields of consciousness embrace all sentient beings, in all times.

From the outset we have focused on some of the most unusual and anomalous experiences imaginable. We took this approach in order to challenge conventional thinking about consciousness and reality and to reveal the much broader expanse of the human spirit. Although many of the experiences covered here may seem to be rare in the context of a modern life-style, within the contexts of energy healing, shamanism and mysticism they are widely known and acknowledged.

People routinely pick up information about the past, hidden, distant and future events with which they have no connection. Conventional thinking, which sees consciousness as an emergent by-product of our neurochemistry, cannot explain this and therefore falls back on denying that such experiences are possible. Nevertheless, many of us access such information on an almost daily basis. It is therefore highly unlikely that consciousness is an emergent property of brain matter. The ability to shift our awareness, for example through empathic engagement with other life forms, maintains perceptual diversity and helps us to holistically relate to the larger web of life. In this way we will naturally be lead in the direction of greater harmony and balance within ourselves, our community and environment.

Meridian therapy techniques (such as Emotional Freedom Techniques and Tapas Acupressure Technique) and rebirthing breathwork, facilitate healing across a broad range of problems. Some of these problems, such as Posttraumatic Stress Disorder, cannot be healed by mainstream medicine. The use of energy therapy techniques reveals aspects of our biographical history that require us to reconsider the limits of consciousness and personal identity. These include memories from our time in the womb. If awareness is 'produced' by the brain then, conventionally speaking, our timeline should only start in the final month before birth when there is enough brain for awareness to arise. What we actually find, however, is that people possess memories that relate to all stages of their fetal life including some memories that are shared with their mother. At the other 'end' of our biographical timeline, we saw that our awareness does not end with death. Numerous near death experiences have been recorded in which people can recall events that they witnessed after they were clinically dead.

In addition, we saw our health and well-being may be deeply influenced by patterns of events 'inherited' from our family and even from ancestors who died long ago. In constellation therapy the emotional tone, the people involved and their individual characteristics become emergent mental, emotional and physical properties of the people representing them. This fact raises a fundamental question as to how and where this information, and its distinctive emotional charge, is stored. Our answer is that it is stored in the larger field of non-local consciousness and not in some complete stranger's brain or DNA. Constellation therapy is only explicable in terms of an unbounded, timeless field of consciousness. It also raises a major question as to how our awareness is capable of decoding this field and restoring the responses of people we never knew and who, in any case, may be long dead. It only requires one of these cases to be true for the conventional understanding of consciousness and reality to be shown to be grossly inadequate.

Rupert Sheldrake's experiments have confirmed the existence of an information bearing and propagating field connected with all sentient life forms that he calls the 'Morphic Field'. In the context of healing we find that people's health and well-being is affected by negative emotional states connected with unresolved family, ancestral and karmic (past life) affects that continue to be propagated through successive generations. Because they are implicated in a majority of cases involving profound healing and personal transformation, we called these fields 'The Healing Field'. They constitute, and are parts of, larger fields of consciousness with which all sentient life forms interact.

In the context of healing, the past is never truly past until it is forgiven. And this connects the operation of these fields with broader issues of agency, meaning and values. Memory is never just neutral information; each memory carries a distinctive emotional charge. When understood it reveals its meaning and embodies a 'spin' or orientation with respect to core values such as justice/injustice, honesty/dishonesty, loyalty/disloyalty and so on. In other words The Healing Field is also an ethical field.

Ancestral and family memories stored within the field directly impinge upon us, whether we are aware of them or not. Just as human awareness is capable of coding and decoding its informational and emotional content, a range of healing modalities demonstrate that it is also possible to recode the field and restore its harmony. Recoding the field involves resolving specific conflicts, injustices and traumas – just as if the people involved where alive and present. This is achieved through a mixture of symbolic re-enactment and the re-establishment of harmony between the 'parties' involved – even if long dead. Harmony is re-established through acknowledging wrongdoing and forgiving transgressions. As a result, operating with the field has a distinctively ethical character. Harmony is associated with such fundamental ethical qualities as justice and respect, and disharmony with the opposing qualities. All of this strongly supports the ancient idea that the field of consciousness, or extended mind, is at root a fundamentally ethical field. It is within our power to recode the field to create ethical congruence and restore harmony. We will return to these ideas in more detail in the next section.

In relation to healing on extended planes of existence, we highlighted the reality of interactions with a broad range of entities of varying degrees of sentience. These entities usually exist in frequency ranges that are invisible to us. They can, however, interact with us positively as well as in ways that undermine our mental, physical and emotional health. On a positive note we explored a range of haunting phenomena that facilitated healing and justice. We also noted that some forms of entity or spirit attachment are positively intentioned. Traumatic experiences can open the energy-body to create a point of ingress that allows entities to attach themselves to it. Such entities are not necessarily hostile. They may identify with that person's problems and seek to help by influencing their thoughts and behavior. Although contacts with otherworldly life-streams can provide instruction and help with healing, when these encounters 'spill over' into the lives of ordinary people, their effects can be deeply disturbing. There is no reason for anyone to feel oppressed by any of these realities. Sufferers can take practical steps to cleanse themselves by simply eliminating the negative emotions and traumas that provide fertile ground for entity attachment. As we saw, the new meridian therapy techniques are perfectly adequate for this purpose.

In the context of healing through spirit, we encountered that ultimate expansion, spiritual or peak experience. At this level of awareness the innately ethical nature of global consciousness becomes self-evident. To have a peak experience is to experience embracing all sentient life with compassion and love. Although such states occur spontaneously, we seldom have the tranquility and psycho-physical preparedness to sustain them. We identified two paths by which systematic work towards their stabilization can be undertaken: the path of pure meditative contemplation and the energized path of excitation or energized meditation. The highest mystical states appear to mark the outer limits of human awareness; they represent the furthest extent to which we can push our awareness. But by focusing on such states simply as another experience to be had, we risk missing their real significance. These higher states act as drivers in the evolutionary unfolding of our innate spiritual potential and contribute towards the healing and harmony of the total web of life. In seeking to realize such states we are following an evolutionary imperative inherent within the nature of the morphic fields underlying all sentient life. Realization implies the dissolution of the limited boundaries of selfhood, boundaries that both define us and our perception of the broader reality. How we experience this dissolution varies greatly from person to person but it is always intrinsically challenging. It is, after all, a foretaste of death itself. All too often discussions of 'realization' attempt to understand it from a purely experiential perspective. What did it feel like? What did you see? This risks missing the essential point of these experiences. Realization is not just a change in perception. It is a change or shift in our entire psychic, energetic and ethical being. It fundamentally changes how we relate to life and death. It shifts our perception of reality from one mediated by intellect to one mediated by the intelligence of the heart. Without this evolutionary shift, peak experiences can be gone just as quickly as they came, leaving regret over their transience, a sense of unworthiness at our inability to sustain or recapture them and a longing for the vision of reality revealed in that one brief moment of realization.

Both excitation and energized mysticism seek to cultivate very high levels of inner energy as the primary vehicle for realizing greatly expanded states of awareness. Needless to say, these practices present certain risks and should not be undertaken casually. Because of the fundamental nature of the shifts involved we urge caution on anyone seeking to explore these highly energized levels of awareness, to make haste slowly, to prepare thoroughly and find experienced supervision. Above all else, balance internal yoga with selfless service in one's community. What these states add to our understanding is a level of comprehension of the larger web of life and of our place within it that overcomes the fear and doubt that are otherwise the lot of the vast majority of humanity.

Consciousness, Evolution & Values

A recent 'meeting of experts asked, 'What would a model of consciousness have to look like that is both true to our modern scientific knowledge and the phenomena reported by spiritual traditions?'[1] The answers that emerged were encapsulated in four main points:

- Consciousness is a fundamental element of reality, like an additional dimension.

- Consciousness is mediated by the brain, not produced by it.

- Consciousness is independent of brain processes.

- Our ability to connect with that which is larger may be a normal state of human beings.

As we have already noted, Sheldrake's concept of the 'Morphic Field', Laszlo's 'A Field' and Mahr's 'Knowing Field' are all consistent with these views. The physicist, Amit Goswami, has usefully summarized Sheldrake's ideas concerning the nature of Morphic Fields in terms of three defining aspects:

a) Teleology. The Morphic, Akashic, Knowing or Healing Field is a purpose driven system. It seeks harmony and therefore ethical congruence.

b) Non-locality. Because the same template serves all of the life-forms who share its structural properties, it is universally available. In other words, the field is accessible everywhere. This is most evident in the context of therapies like Family Constellations where complete strangers are unconsciously able to access and model the behavior, thoughts and emotions of individuals involved in family and ancestral conflicts despite the fact that they have no prior knowledge of the people or issues involved.

c) Downward causation. Through a process Sheldrake has called 'morphic resonance', the field propagates its effects to all of its members.

To these points we can now add the following three:

- The field of consciousness (whether on the personal, family or ancestral levels) is sensitive to the harmony and disharmony that arise in connection with the ethical quality of our actions.

- The fact that emotional disharmony persists in a multi-generational way and is capable of impacting our health and well-being, confirms that consciousness must be a pervasive morphic field.

- The field is coded, decoded and recoded, and therefore (ethically) reharmonized, using defocalized awareness, symbolic enactment and ethical rebalancing. This itself is astonishing, and brings a different perspective to discussions of consciousness and reality.

The introduction of ethical considerations points towards the larger role of ethical behavior in the evolutionary unfolding of all sentient life. Put bluntly, harmonious action (expressed through such positive qualities as fairness, justice, loyalty, freedom and respect) equals health, healing and spiritual growth. Disharmonious action, based upon the opposite qualities, halts or even reverses this. We noted the 'civilizing function' of the higher initiations, such as those associated with the Bwiti religion and the ancient mysteries. These institutions were designed to facilitate a shift in awareness that enabled the initiates to view themselves, their communities and all sentient life as integral parts of the web of life. The result of this experience of the essential unity and continuity of all life is a greatly expanded understanding, tolerance and compassion. Such shifts fundamentally affect a permanent relativization of the egoic self and allow us to occupy a higher ground with respect to our humanity.

These levels of realization represent an upward moving, expansive impulse that is inherent in all sentient beings. When stabilized, such awareness facilitates higher orders of behavior that manifest evolutionarily higher orders of values. Values are an inherent aspect of both human and animal behavior. As we will see their manifestation in different societies and cultures demonstrates a deep and consistent structure.

Values

The arc of the moral universe is long, but it bends towards justice

Martin Luther King Jr.

In recent years a leading moral philosopher, Alistair MacIntyre, has claimed, "We have – very largely, if not entirely – lost our comprehension, both theoretical and practical, of morality".[2] However we interpret this, it certainly appears as though we face a crisis of values. If nothing else, globalization has led to a collision of cultures, beliefs and values. But long before the era of globalization, from the 18th century onwards, modernity experienced its own crisis of values. Ethics has not fared well amongst modernist intellectual elites. On the one hand, moral judgments have been declared to be no more than random sounds of personal approval or disapproval (Emotivism). On the other, many modern thinkers, from Jeremy Bentham to Ayn Rand, treat values as systems for the rational optimization of benefits, whether for the larger community (Utilitarianism) or for one's own private ends (Egoism). These abstract, intellectual conceptions are quite remote from lived experience. At root, values are something that we feel in our innermost being. These moral feelings quite literally shape our experience of reality, directing our attention towards or away from what is happening around us. As the philosopher, John McMurtry, summarized it, "we might best understand our human reality as a vast and complex field of values"[3]. Recent research by psychologist

Jonathan Haidt has helped to clarify the extent to which values are fundamental to life[4]:

They possess intuitive primacy – people have nearly instant reactions to scenes or stories of moral violations. Affective reactions are usually good predictors of moral judgments and behaviors.

They guide social behavior – when we believe that something is 'right' we are naturally inclined to act in a way that is consistent with this feeling.

They bind and build community – morality constrains individuals and ties them to each other to create groups. A moral community has a set of shared norms about how members ought to behave.

Where and how does this sense of 'intuitive primacy' arise? Based upon the direct evidence that we have already cited, it is clear that The Healing Field that connects us to one another, to our family and ancestral past and to the wider community of all sentient life, is a moral field that exerts a 'pressure' for right action and the correction of past wrongs. There is nothing new about this insight. In fact it is one of the most ancient conceptions of ethics known to us. Some 2,400 years ago Aristotle described values as 'right by nature'. Values are an integral part of the fabric of reality, at once absolute and universal but at the same time variable and localized,

"that which everywhere has the same force and does not exist by people's thinking this or that … and yet all of it is changeable"[5]

But if values are integral to and emergent from the fabric of reality, if they impart a positive force for right action and the correction of past wrongs – in short, for justice – what implications does this have for us and how we live our lives?

Integral Theory

The insight that values drive the progressive social and spiritual evolution of all sentient life occurred simultaneously to a number of thinkers around the turn of the 20th century. In particular Sri Aurobindo, Rudolph Steiner, Pitirim Sorokin and Jean Gebser contributed towards elucidating these ideas, a body of thought called 'Integral Theory'. In the 1950s the social psychologist Claire Graves undertook research that placed many of these ideas on a firmer basis, "Briefly, what I am proposing is that the psychology of the mature human being is an unfolding, emergent, oscillating spiraling process marked by progressive subordination of older, lower-order behavior systems to newer, higher-order systems as man's existential problems change."[6] More recently Graves' work has received confirmation from that of anthropologist Richard Shweder. A comparative analysis of moral discourse across cultures reveals that all moral discourse 'fits into' one of three fundamental sets of values[7]:

Ethics of autonomy, based upon such concepts as harm, rights, fairness and justice.

Ethics of community, based upon duty, hierarchy, tradition, respect and loyalty.

Ethics of divinity, based upon sacred order, sanctity, purity and sin.

Graves recognized that our moral responses manifest with a greater or lesser degree of sophistication that represents an evolutionary factor in the unfolding of human consciousness[8]. By modulating our responses to the challenges that we are faced with in the light of our most evolved set of values we enable healing, integration and transformation to take place personally, societally and globally.

This evolutionary unfolding of consciousness is being played out across the entire planet. Regressive forces, such as threats to survival, whether real or imagined, can drive entire societies to enact earlier, more primitive patterns of behavior. And herein lays a great danger. Threats to our survival, whether real or imagined, can be manipulated to mobilize people for wars that are waged to benefit certain sectional interests. One side effect of these social eruptions, apart from the injuries and loss of life they entail, is a reversal of our evolutionary progress. It is possible for a society to stagnate ethically when the majority of its people become disconnected from their natural sense of community and are encouraged to inhabit a distorted and distorting view of themselves, others and of reality itself. The development of Graves' ideas into the conflict-resolution system called 'Spiral Dynamics'[9] emphasizes the fact that only evolutionarily higher orders of ethical behavior are able to solve the increasingly complex issues facing us today.

Recent research has highlighted the relative lack of empathy amongst many of the people who aspire to the highest positions of leadership in any society. This implies that we can come to be led by people who share few, if any, of the core values of humanity[10,11,12]. Across the globe the leading edge of societal and spiritual evolution, the so-called 'cultural creatives'[13], are actively engaged in co-creating the future by re-sculpting their lives based on a foundation of personal and spiritual development, social equality, environmental awareness and responsible consumption. The emerging global society is being shaped, slowly but surely, by fundamentally ethical concerns. This translates into, amongst other things, a respect for all forms of diversity, including the perceptual diversity of altered states. In the light of this it is incumbent upon each and every one of us to demonstrate leadership by taking responsibility for the quality of life in our own communities. Too many of us imagine that the spiritual path is one of meditation in an isolated cave hidden away in some remote mountains. But when we realize that we are all, quite literally, connected, and actively engaged, whether mindfully or not, in co-creating and maintaining the ethical quality of the fields that connect us, then healing, personal development and spiritual practices must be extended into the communities that we live in. For this to be possible profound processes of healing are required at all levels of society. Each and every one of us needs to sit up and take notice of the way that modernity is currently structured. For it has been designed to distract our attention from reality and direct it towards an imaginary and, in many cases, highly negative world view.

Modernity is an altered state of consciousness

"We must shift ... from a needs to a desires culture. People must be trained to desire, to want new things, even before the old have been entirely consumed ... Man's desires must overshadow his needs."[14]

It will no doubt strike the reader as odd to find 'modernity', immersion in a consumer hyper-reality, described as an altered state, but that is exactly what it is. The mass democracies that emerged in the early 20th century out of the processes of industrialization created new challenges for traditional mechanisms of political, economic and social control. One response to these challenges has been to engage in the mass manipulation of awareness, the engineering of consent[15], through propaganda and the manipulation of desire via the mass media (for example by advertising, product placement, and the promotion of aspirational 'life-styles'),

"The conscious and intelligent manipulation of the organized habits and opinions of the masses is an important element in democratic society. Those who manipulate this unseen mechanism of society constitute an invisible government which is the true ruling power of our country."[16]

This manipulation of desire hinges upon the creation of a gap between media projected ideals and each person's imagined progress towards their realization. It is, essentially, a manipulation and falsification of self-concept designed to trigger the kinds of behavior – engagement with financial and market mechanisms – that provide a temporary sense of 'completeness'. We are guided to realize this temporary sense of completeness through the acquisition of products and services that have been prepositioned and promoted fetishized as defining the various aspects of an idealized and narcisstic image of selfhood beauty, strength, competence, superiority, mastery and so on. The pervasiveness of media controlled images and the celebrity culture that mediates this process has created societies driven by greed, distracted by trivia and in thrall to spectacle[17], even when that spectacle includes the destruction of other peoples. To these sources of distortion we can add environmental, pharmacological and electromagnetic pollution on a massive scale; the manipulation of mood via entertainment, food additives and a whole range of narcotics, whether legitimate or otherwise. Modernity, the typical form of consciousness emerging from the confluence of these forces, itself constitutes a potent altered state. It is designed to leave us stranded in 'hyper-reality' – were reality and fantasy become indistinguishable or where reality is dispensed with altogether in favor of fantasy[18].

It is self-evident that such conditions tend to undermine, if not reverse, the evolutionary process identified by Graves as the "subordination of older, lower-order behavior systems to newer, higher-order systems". In other words, as humanity, we are faced with a direct threat to our ethical and spiritual evolution. Recognizing that the modes of awareness arising out of modernity are dead ends engendering potent altered states of self-absorbed fantasy, what can we do to re-establish our relationship with the broader, evolutionary field of spiritualized awareness?

What can we do?

> *Want the change. Be inspired by the flame where*
> *everything shines as it disappears*
>
> *Rilke, Sonnets to Orpheus, Part II, XII*

The opposite of living immersed in a consumer hyper-reality is to live 'authentically'. But what does this mean? No doubt it means something different for every person. I would like to suggest that however we realize it, it involves accepting complete and unconditional responsibility for each and every aspect of the quality of our own experience. Please note, I did not say accepting responsibility, for example, for our lot in life or how society is structured and operates. I said taking responsibility for the quality of our own experience. This task operates alongside, not instead of, efforts to reform out of date political, economic and social structures.

The challenge that we are addressing is to improve the quality of our own experience by realizing positive shifts in our psycho-energetic being. The foundation for achieving this is through emotional integration. We can start by identifying every aspect of our experience that disturbs us and commit ourselves to changing our relationship to it by changing ourselves. The question of our relationship with those aspects of reality that we find most distasteful, or most addictive, is one of the subtlest and most complex of issues. And yet experience overwhelmingly demonstrates that there is an intimate relationship between how we are in our innermost being and the quality of our lived experience. This relationship is such that when we change ourselves we change our relationship with reality and this provides us with the leverage to re-sculpt our lives. The question then becomes, what is the nature of the change that we seek? How do we ensure that it aligns with fundamental values and supports the spiritual evolution of all sentient beings?

The starting place of ancient ethics was the search for 'eudemonia', roughly, 'the good life'. In recent years positive psychology has undertaken the job of 'unpacking' these ancient ideas and providing them with a scientific foundation. Eudemonia is usually translated as 'human flourishing' and its benefits positively impact every single area of life without exception[19,20].

Most of us associate, or in the past have associated, happiness with external circumstances – with becoming 'better off'. And yet such 'happiness', like a mirage, always seems to recede in front of us. Studies have demonstrated that external circumstances play a very small part, around 10%-15%, in our overall levels of happiness. Fully half of our capacity for happiness is thought to be determined by relatively fixed factors that constitute our 'set-point' or baseline level of happiness to which we return after experiencing any high point. This only leaves around one third of our capacity for happiness susceptible to intentional activity[21]. Clearly our 'set point' or baseline level of happiness accounts for the majority of our reactions to life's ups and downs. Other circumstances, factors such as age, gender, education and income, appear to have only a marginal impact. The question therefore is, is it possible to increase our overall levels of happiness? We need to split this question into two parts:

- Firstly, what 'inner work' do we need to undertake to overcome the inertia of our 'set-point' and shift our baseline level of happiness in a positive direction?

- Secondly, how should we manage our intentional activity to optimize eudemonia, our happiness and flourishing?

Overturning the set-point

We noted in Chapter 3 (Healing) that consciousness exhibits a multi-layered continuum that includes perinatal memory, past lives, family and ancestral influences. We can use this structure to guide our inner work. Apart from our immediate senses and memory, we remain largely unconscious of the other layers. The only way that we can assess the work required in each of these layers is by paying careful attention to our moment to moment experience. How often do we find ourselves lost in negative thoughts and feelings? What is the ratio of our negative to positive thoughts and feelings? What is the quality of our 'self-talk'? Are there certain 'tracks', narratives of self-blame and criticism, that we constantly play to ourselves over and over again? Are there also certain negative recurrent patterns manifesting in our relationships with loved ones or those in authority? By starting with these most mundane, and yet most persistent, of concerns we can begin to expand our self-awareness and this is the prelude to enhancing self-management. To enact self-management we should identify and master a small number of easy to use, self-empowering techniques and practices. The new meridian therapies and a basic skill with mindfulness are excellent candidates for this. It is essential, however, that we always seek to achieve the complete integration of any issue that draws our attention. For example, at the level of our present moment awareness and biographical memory we can utilize the various energy psychology techniques to eliminate specific negative thoughts and feelings and replace them with positive ones. For particularly deep issues we may seek to establish a 'buddy' system or get some sessions from an experienced professional. The clearing of these 'presenting' issues can, and often does, lead to the clearing of issues at much deeper levels, including birth related (perinatal), past life and family/ancestral issues. Working directly at these deeper, unconscious levels can be undertaken by utilizing techniques that employ very high levels of inner energy such as Rebirthing Breathwork. Initially, rebirthing breathwork needs to be supervised by an experienced practitioner. During these sessions we should never try to 'push' ourselves too hard. It is essential with such techniques to always remain within one's comfort zone. Rebirthing breathwork can be very intense and is not for everyone. Focusing on the deeper layers of consciousness we may want to explore past lives. It is not unusual for traumatic deaths in past lives to be 'carried forward' into this life, manifesting in a variety of physical, mental and emotional conditions that defy explanation and resolution but which are readily dissolved once the traumatic experience of a previous death is integrated. Past life regression therapy provides a good venue for this activity. Inherited ancestral influences affecting us in this life can be resolved through such systems as Family Constellations Therapy. Always find facilitators through positive referral, they should have good reputations for empathy, compassion and skill.

In parallel with the clearing of blockages to the free flow of our life-energy, we should seek to develop our capacity for mindfulness through regular meditative practice. An enhanced capacity for stilling the mind and being comfortable with stillness is essential to break many of the addictive patterns that distract us from ourselves and what is really happening around us. Mindfulness also opens up the space for us to 'tune in' and receive the subtle information that is available in the broader field of consciousness.

Apart from our program of 'inner work', we all need to look at the texture of our day to day lives. A useful framework that we can all adopt suggests that human flourishing arises from the managed convergence of three related life strategies: the Pleasant Life, or life of enjoyment, the Good Life, or life of engagement, and the Meaningful Life, or life of affiliation[22].

The 'Pleasant Life' consists of simply having as many pleasurable experiences as possible. Few of us would want to object to this idea, and with good reason. Unsurprisingly, as a life strategy this approach doesn't lead to a stable sense of personal fulfillment or enduring happiness. It has been found that after some months even lottery winners revert to much the same (and sometimes an even worse) emotional state than before they won the lottery.[23] From an early age most of us are, to some degree, addicted to the 'Pleasant Life'. It is, after all, the force that drives consumerism. But its satisfactions are, inevitably, transitory. The evaporation of the emotional 'high' associated with new experiences leaves us once more face to face with ourselves – our 'raw' state of being – or 'set-point' to which we return again and again. When pursued to the exclusion of all else, the 'Pleasant Life' is also the 'Dissatisfied Life'. Boredom drives an endless search for new sources of stimulation. Fortunately, this is not the only strategy open to us. If we enjoy our pleasures and yet remain unfulfilled, then we need to look to the next level – to the 'good life'.

The 'Good Life' involves deep engagement in work, family life or any other activities that give rise to a profound sense of personal satisfaction and fulfillment. All of the available research agrees that our relationships with our family and friends are one of the most important contributors to our overall levels of happiness. Parallel with these relationships are all of the other areas of life with which we are involved. In particular our work lives absorb a large amount of our waking hours. To engage deeply with something we need to be able to identify and then apply our greatest strengths & capabilities, sometimes known as 'signature strengths'[24], to it. Utilizing our most defining strengths and capabilities gives rise to a profound sense of well-being that is anchored in the deepest levels of our being. Applying yourself completely to something that fully engages your strengths typically leads to a state of complete absorption called 'flow'[25]. Flow is a state that people experience when they are completely absorbed in what they are doing to the point of forgetting time, fatigue, and everything else but what they are doing. The experience of flow has been described as "being completely involved in an activity for its own sake. The ego falls away. Time flies. Every action, movement, and thought follows inevitably from the previous one, like playing jazz. Your whole being is involved, and you're using your skills to the utmost."[26] If you have never or only infrequently experience flow, then you probably need to check what your signature strengths are[27], look at how you are using them on a day to day basis and begin to re-sculpt your life to engage more of your strengths more fully more of the time. But even attaining the 'Good or Engaged Life' may still not provide the sense of purpose & fulfillment that we seek, "just as well-being needs to be anchored in strengths & virtues, these in turn must be anchored in something larger. Just as the good life is something beyond the pleasant life, the meaningful life is beyond the good life."[28]

The 'Meaningful Life' consists in placing our signature strengths in the service of a cause larger than our selves. We derive a positive sense of well-being, belonging, meaning, and purpose from being part of and contributing to something larger and more permanent (e.g. nature, charity/community groups, organizations, movements, and belief systems). One area in which these higher levels of engagement emerge is 'authentic leadership'. Major life challenges have the potential to generate an inner transformation characterized as moving from an 'I' to a 'We' perspective[29], a shift in orientation from service to self to service to others. Moving from focusing on one's own private goals and targets to taking responsibility for a collective and for serving its goals and objectives, even at personal cost, has been called "entering the fundamental state of leadership".[30] It is characterized as moving:

- moving beyond one's comfort zone to explore new possibilities
- acting from one's core values rather than conforming to other's expectations
- acting for the collective good rather than pursuing self-interest
- embracing change rather than relying on routines

On this planet we are faced with enormous challenges but through these we can see, if only dimly, the outlines of a future humanity existing on a higher arc of spiritual evolution. The task of realizing this future is not someone else's. It is certainly not the task of the some remote political or corporate elite. The task of realizing this better future is yours, and mine, and all of us who wish for something better not only for ourselves and our loved ones, but for all sentient life and who grasp the fact that we are, all of us, a part of a greater whole.

"A person experiences life as something separated from the rest - a kind of optical delusion of consciousness. Our task must be to free ourselves from this self-imposed prison, and through compassion, to find the reality of Oneness."

Albert Einstein

Notes

1. Forman, R. 'A Watershed Event: Neuroscience, Consciousness and Spirituality Conference', July 2–4, 2008, Freiburg Germany' Journal of Consciousness Studies, 15, No. 8, 2008, pp. 110–15

2. MacIntyre, A. (1984) After Virtue: A Study in Moral Theory p. 1-5.

3. McMurtry, J. 'The Global Crisis of Values'

4. Haidt, J. 'The New Synthesis in Moral Psychology' Science, Volume 316, 998 (2007)

5. Aristotle Nichomachean Ethics Book V 1134bl8-20.

6. Graves, C. (1974) 'Human Nature Prepares for a Momentus Leap' The Futurist, April 1974 p.72-87

7. Shweder, RA., Much, NC., Mahapatra, M., & Park, L. (1997) 'The "big three" of morality and the "big three" explanations of suffering' in Brandt, AM. & Rozin, P. (Editors) (1997) Morality and Health (pp. 119–169)

8. Graves, C. 'Human Nature Prepares for a Momentous Leap' The Futurist, April 1974, p.72-87

9. Beck, D. & Cowan, C. (1996) Spiral Dynamics: Mastering Values, Leadership and Change

10. Piff, PK. et al 'Having less, giving more: The influence of social class on prosocial behavior' Journal of Personality and Social Psychology, Volume: 99(5), Nov 2010, 771-784

11. Kraus, M., Cote, S., & Keltner, D. 'Social Class, Contextualism, and Empathic Accuracy' Psychological Science, 2010, 21 (11), 1716-1723

12. Boar, BJ. & Fritzon, K. 'Disordered Personalities at Work' Psychology, Crime & Law, March 2005, Vol. 11(1)

13. Ray, PH. & Anderson, SR. (2000) The Cultural Creatives: How 50 Million People Are Changing the World

14. *Wall Street banker Paul Mazur from the 1930s, cited in Adam Curtis' documentary 'The Century of the Self'*

15. *Bernays, EL. (1947) 'The Engineering of Consent', Annals of the American Academy of Political and Social Science, 250 p. 113.*

16. *Bernays, EL. (1928) Propaganda p.1*

17. *Debord, G. (1967) The Society of the Spectacle*

18. *Baudrillard, J. (1981) Simulacra and Simulation*

19. *Fredrickson, B 'The Broaden & Build Theory of Positive Emotions' Philosophical Transactions of the Royal Society, August 2004*

20. *Fredrickson, B & Losada, MF 'Positive Affect & the Complex Dynamics of Human Flourishing' American Psychologist, October 2005*

21. *Lyubomirsky, Sheldon & Schanke'Pusuing Happiness: The Architectuire of Sustainable Change' Review of general Psychology, 2005, Vol. 9, No. 2, 111–131*

22. *Seligman, M. (2005) Authentic Happiness: Using the New Positive Psychology to Realize Your Potential for Lasting Fulfilment*

23. *Brickman, P., Coates, D. & Janoff-Bulman, R. 'Lottery winners and accident victims: is happiness relative?', Journal of Personality and Social Psychology, 1978, 36, 8: 917-927.*

24. *Seligman, M. & Peterson, C. 'Character Strengths and Virtues: A Handbook and Classification'*

25. *Csikszentmihalyi, M. 'Flow: The Psychology of Optimal Experience', 1990*

26. *'Go With the Flow' Wired Magazine, Issue 4.09, Sep 1996*

27. *VIA Signature Strengths Survey is available online at www. authentichappiness.com*

28. *Seligman, M (2005) op cit. p.14*

29. George, W. & McLean, A. 'The Transformation From I to We' *Leader to Leader* (spring 2007)

30. Quinn, RE. 'Moments of Greatness: Entering the Fundamental State of Leadership' *Harvard Business Review*, July-August 2005

Bibliography

Aristotle 'Nichomachean Ethics'

Ayer, AJ. (1956) The Problem of Knowledge

Baldwin, WJ. & Fiore, E. (1995) Spirit Releasement Therapy: A Technique Manual

Beck, D. & Cowan, C. (1996) Spiral Dynamics: Mastering Values, Leadership, and Change

Bernays, E. (1928) Propaganda

Burkert, W. (1987) Ancient Mystery Cults

Cicero 'On the Laws'

Csikszentmihalyi, M. (1990) Flow: The Psychology of Optimal Experience

Debord, G. (1967) The Society of the Spectacle

Fermor, PL. (1957) A Time to Keep Silence

Fiore, E. (1987) The Unquiet Dead: A Psychologist Treats Spirit Possession

Foucault, M. (2005) The Hermeneutics of the Subject: Lectures at the College de France 1981-82

Grof, S. (1992) The Holotropic Mind: The Three Levels of Human Consciousness & How They Shape Our Lives

Grof, S. & C. (eds.) (1989) Spiritual Emergencies: When Personal Transformation Becomes a Crisis

Hadot, P. (1995) Philosophy as a Way of Life: spiritual exercises from Socrates to Foucault

Happold, HC. (1963) Mysticism

Hellinger, B. (1998) Love's Hidden Symmetry: what makes love work in relationships

James, W. (1902) The Varieties of Religious Experience

Kauffman, S. (2008) Reinventing the Sacred: A New View of Science, Reason, and Religion

Kerenyi, K. (1967) Eleusis: Archetypal Image of Mother and Daughter

Krippner, S. 'Altered States of Consciousness' in J. White (Editor) (1972) The Highest State of Consciousness

Lewis-Williams, DJ. (2002) The Mind In The Cave: Consciousness and the Origins of Art

MacIntyre, A. (1984) After Virtue: A Study in Moral Theory

Maslow, AH. (1964) Religions, Values and Peak Experiences

Merton, T. (1978) The New Man

Miller, H. (2002) Dowsing: a Journey Beyond Our Senses

Modi, Dr. S. (1998) Remarkable Healings: A Psychiatrist Discovers Unsuspected Roots of Mental and Physical Illness

Nagel, T. (2012) Mind and Cosmos: Why the Materialist Neo-Darwinian Conception of Nature is Almost Certainly False

Nan, Huai-Chin Nan (1984) Tao and Longevity: Mind-Body Transformation

Oschman, JL. (2000) Energy Medicine: The Scientific Basis

Plato Theaetetus 201b-d.

Sagan, S. (1994) Entity Possession: Freeing the Energy-body of Negative Influences

Seligman, M. (2005) Authentic Happiness: Using the New Positive Psychology to Realize Your Potential for Lasting Fulfilment

Sheldrake, R. (1988) The Presence of the Past: Morphic Resonance and the Habits of Nature

Sheldrake, R. (2009) Morphic Resonance: The Nature of Formative Causation

Sinclair, A. (1993) The Sword and the Grail

Sogyal Rinpoche (1992) The Tibetan Book of Living and Dying

Tao Te Ching

Tart, CT. (ed.) (1969) 'Altered States of Consciousness: A Book of Readings'

Taylor, C. (2007) A Secular Age

Underhill, E. (1911) Mysticism: A Study of the Nature and Development of Man's Spiritual Consciousness

Vaughan, H. (1905) The Poems of Henry Vaughan Silurist

Wong, E. (trans.) Hui Ming Ching (The Book of Consciousness and Life)

Index

About the Author

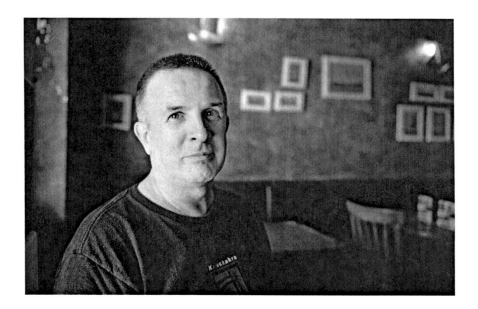

Peter Mark Adams, a Philosophy graduate, has been researching energy, consciousness and healing for over 35 years. For the past 20 years he has worked as a professional rebirthing breathwork facilitator, mindfulness teacher, energy therapist, Usui Reiki teacher and author.

Peter has written a range of practical manuals covering Mindfulness, Reiki and Rebirthing Breathwork. He has contributed numerous articles on complementary and alternative medicine, mindfulness, Reiki, breathwork, energy, esotericism and altered states of consciousness to a range of journals. Peter is a contributor to Paranthropology, the international peer reviewed journal of anthropological approaches to the paranormal and 'The Journal of Exceptional Experiences and Psychology'. Peter has acted as both an advisor and contributor to the Turkish Radio & Television documentary 'On the Borders of Science'.

For over 15 years Peter and his wife, Gulcan, have been practising energy healing and teaching thousands of people. Gulcan, an industrial engineer, specialises in emotional and karmic healing. This book is a testimony to their teamwork. They live in Istanbul with a cocker spaniel and three cats.

Peter can be contacted through his web site:
www.petermarkadams.com

CPSIA information can be obtained at www.ICGtesting.com
Printed in the USA
LVOW11s1800100914

403444LV00001B/265/P